Stop

Depression

Now

RICHARD BROWN, M.D.

TEODORO BOTTIGLIERI, PH.D.

CAROL COLMAN

G.P. Putnam's Sons
New York

Stop Depression Now

SAM-e

*The Breakthrough Supplement
That Works As Well
As Presciption Drugs
in Half the Time...
with No Side Effects*

G. P. Putnam's Sons
Publishers Since 1838
a member of
Penguin Putnam Inc.
375 Hudson Street
New York, NY 10014

Library of Congress Cataloging-in-Publication Data

Brown, Richard, date.
Stop depression now: SAM-e, the breakthrough
supplement that works as well as prescription drugs
in half the time, with no side effects / Richard Brown,
Teodoro Bottiglieri, Carol Colman.
p.   cm.
Includes bibliographical references.
ISBN 0-399-14530-3 (alk. paper)
1. Depression, Mental—Alternative treatment.
2. Depression, Mental—Chemotherapy.
I. Bottiglieri, Teodoro.   II. Colman, Carol.
III. Title.
RC537.B765   1999   99-27451   CIP
616.85'27061—dc21

Printed in the United States of America
1   3   5   7   9   10   8   6   4   2

This book is printed on acid-free paper. ∞

Book design by Deborah Kerner

Acknowledgments

Many people helped with this book. First and foremost, we would like to thank our editor, Jeremy Katz, for his extraordinarily hard work and creative vision. Without him, this book simply would not have happened. We would also like to thank the dedicated team at Penguin Putnam who made this book a reality in record time, including Tricia Martin, Catharine Lynch, Diane Lomonaco, Ann Spinelli, Lisa Amoroso, Coral Tysliava, Elizabeth Wagner, Claire Vaccaro, Marilyn Ducksworth, and Fern Edison.

Much thanks to Dr. Robert Spitzer for giving us permission to use his depression severity scale. Our thanks as well to Dr. Giorgio Stramentinoli for his seminal research on SAM-e. We would also like to thank Meg Schneider and Jo Sgammato for their help and support.

To Pat for the help and patience

— RB

To Gisela, Marco and Alesio

— TB

To Michael and Josh

— CC

Author's Note

SAM-e is a remarkable substance and a boon to depression therapy. However, it is not a complete cure for all depressions. Because of depression's complexities and its myriad presentations, there is no single drug that is a total cure for everyone. Nevertheless, SAM-e is one of the best weapons we have in the fight against depression.

On average, SAM-e begins to relieve depression in seven days, although some people may need more time. Most prescription drugs take two to four weeks or more to show results. It is important to remember that your experience may vary, but as a general rule, SAM-e starts working in half the time (or less) than is needed for prescription antidepressants.

No substance has absolutely no side effects: if researchers were to perform a clinical trial on water, they would likely receive reports of any number of adverse reactions. SAM-e comes about as close to no side effects as you can get. In clinical trials, it caused fewer side effects than a placebo—a sugar pill. At high doses—doses much higher than any we recommend in this book—a few people complain of mild, transient headache, loose bowels (probably due to bile being released from the liver, and usually relieved by fiber), or overstimulation (similar to the effects of caffeine), which soon disappears. Patients prone to panic disorder can react to even tiny doses of any antidepressant with some anxiety, and this is true of SAM-e. However, if SAM-e causes these side effects, they are usually much milder, briefer, and more easily tolerated than side effects caused by other antidepressants. Although bipolar patients may become manic on any effective antidepressant and may develop mild, brief hypomania on SAM-e, SAM-e may still be helpful for patients with bipolar depression in low doses with mood stabilizers and under the supervision by an experienced psychiatrist. Again, your experience may vary.

Contents

Stop

Depression

Now

———

Part I

The Safe, Fast, New Way to Beat Depression

1

Stop Depression Now

You *don't* have to be depressed.

You don't have to see a doctor and wait for him or her to write you a prescription.

You don't have to suffer the miserable side effects of standard prescription antidepressants.

You don't have to endure weeks or months of waiting for your antidepressant drug to start working.

You can stop your depression *right now.* In fact, you can feel much better in a matter of just days.

And you can find all the tools you need to conquer your depression quickly and safely right here in these pages.

Stop Depression Now will introduce you to a break-through supplement called SAM-e (pronounced "sammy") that is revolutionizing the treatment of depression and is about to change the lives of the millions of Americans battling this ailment. SAM-e—scientific shorthand for S-adenosyl-methionine—has been widely available in Europe for more than two decades, but is only now being sold in the United States. You can find it over the counter at pharmacies, natural food stores, discount department store chains, and supermarkets.

At this very moment, some 17 million Americans suffer from clinical, diagnosed depression, a chronic and potentially life-threatening condition. About one in eight Americans—some twenty-five percent of all women and twelve percent of all men—are diagnosed with serious depression at some point in their lives.

Many more will suffer in silence. Depression all too often goes undetected and untreated. Researchers estimate that as many as half of all people who endure this condition never seek medical attention. The numbers are staggering. Depression is no less an epidemic than heart disease or cancer. In fact, depression is the number one ailment physicians are called upon to diagnose and treat.

The majority of people with clinical depression experience mild-to-moderate symptoms. Their depression may not prevent them from carrying out life's pressing responsibilities, but it does stand in the way of their enjoying a rich, fulfilling life. *Stop Depression Now* speaks to people whose depression interferes with their ability to have the kind of life they want to live.

But maybe you are not clinically depressed. Maybe you simply don't have as bright an outlook as you could. Or maybe you have "the blues" or just some persistent unhappiness. Increasingly, doctors and patients alike have begun to recognize that these symptoms—lumped together in a class called subsyndromal depression—cause real suffering and have real impact on people's lives. This is the gray zone—an area of little medical attention. A feeling of colorlessness in life, the gray zone does not include bad moods, lousy days, or even an occasional funk. No, people in the gray zone just feel *down*—not every day, but often enough to wonder what's wrong.

Although SAM-e is new to the United States, it is not untried or untested. Quite the contrary. It is currently being used by more than a million Europeans. For more than three decades, SAM-e has been the subject of literally thousands of scientific studies conducted at the world's leading research centers, including Harvard Medical School, the University of California, and King's College Hospital in London. Moreover, dozens of articles in leading medical journals around the world have featured SAM-e. SAM-e is the only natural supplement to undergo such rigorous scientific research. So solid is the research that SAM-e has been approved for use as a *prescription* drug in Spain, Italy, Russia, and Germany. Indeed, in Italy, SAM-e outsells the antidepressant Prozac, despite the fact that for technical reasons, Italian insurance companies will reimburse only for Prozac. When given the choice, people are opting to take SAM-e over Prozac, even though they have to pay extra for it!

Study after study has confirmed that SAM-e works as well as or better than any other antidepressant. Studies show that it works faster, often in a matter of days, while other antidepressants may take weeks or even months to kick in. Amazingly, SAM-e takers experience virtually no side effects, whereas side effects constitute one of the major problems with every other antidepressant, including St. John's wort. Indeed, there is compelling evidence that SAM-e is useful in treating other conditions as well, and may just become the treatment of choice not only for depression but also for osteoarthritis and fibromyalgia. In other words, SAM-e has no side effects . . . only side benefits.

Unlike other antidepressants, SAM-e is not a drug. Nor is it an herb or even a vitamin. Rather, it is a substance normally produced by every living organism on the planet, including human beings. This is one of the big differences between taking SAM-e and using any other antidepressant, such as Prozac or even the herb St. John's wort. With prescription antidepressants or their herbal counterparts, you are introducing a foreign chemical into your body. When you take SAM-e, you are merely supplementing something that is already present in every cell. Perhaps SAM-e works so well and so harmoniously because it belongs in our bodies in the first place. It restores the mind and body to the state at which they function best.

But before we get any farther, allow me to tell you who we are and why we feel this book is so ground-breaking and important.

My name is Richard Brown, M.D. I am an associate professor of clinical psychiatry at Columbia University College of Physicians and Surgeons in New York City. I am a mainstream, traditionally trained psychiatrist with private practices in New York City and the up-state New York rural community where I live. Much of my career has been spent as a research physician in an academic environment, where I have participated in a number of scientific studies on the treatment of psychiatric disorders. Like a growing number of physicians today, I employ both conventional prescription drugs and alternative therapies in my practice. I consider myself open-minded, yet I do not recommend any treatment—be it prescription medication, herb, or any other type of therapy—unless there is a sound scientific basis for it. I am a stickler for good science. If the science isn't there, I will not recommend a treatment. As I explain to my patients, just because a product is "natural" doesn't necessarily mean it is safe or effective. Nature is filled with wonderful medicines that can heal, and also potent poisons that can kill. It is important to know the difference.

I have been using SAM-e in my practice for more than five years. It has been extremely difficult, until now, to obtain SAM-e in the United States, and my patients have gone to great lengths—literally—to get it. Some have actually made trips to Europe solely for the

purpose of buying SAM-e. Others have implored over-
seas relatives to send it to them, at great cost, or have
purchased it from offshore suppliers who could not
guarantee timely delivery or quality control. Given
what some of my patients have had to go through to
get SAM-e, I am delighted that a high-quality form of
SAM-e is now at last readily available in the United
States.

My coauthor, Teodoro (Terry) Bottiglieri, Ph.D., is
a senior research scientist and director of neuropharmacology at Baylor University Medical Center's Institute of Metabolic Diseases, Mass Spectrometry, and
Biochemical Diagnostic Unit, in Dallas, Texas, as well
as an associate professor at the university. Born and
educated in England, Terry did his Ph.D. thesis on
SAM-e more than fifteen years ago and has been studying it ever since. He's dedicated his entire career to the
science of SAM-e, and although he is too modest to
say so himself, Terry is a superb researcher and one of
the world's leading authorities on SAM-e. If you scan
the bibliography at the back of this book, you will see
that Terry has coauthored many of the groundbreaking
studies on SAM-e. In addition, he is an internationally
acclaimed expert on the role of nutrition in depression,
a topic that we cover later in the book, in Chapter 7
("The Stop Depression Now Food Plan"). Some of you
may already be familiar with the link between two B
vitamins—folic acid and B_{12}—in treating mood disorders. What you probably do not know is that Terry

was instrumental in discovering this connection. Long before I met Terry in person, I followed his research and was well aware of his contributions to this new field.

Terry and I are writing this book to share our knowledge and experience with SAM-e with both laypeople and physicians. Terry's work on SAM-e and the biology of depression has provided the scientific basis for the book and a goodly chunk of what science knows about this supplement. I, on the other hand, am a psychopharmacologist, a subspeciality of psychiatry. I no longer work in the lab and instead spend my time treating patients. As a psychopharmacologist, I treat the biological as well as the psychological components of mental disorders, of which depression is the most common by far.

Some people may believe that depression should only be treated by a psychiatrist, and that it is wrong to encourage people to use an over-the-counter treatment like SAM-e. I disagree. But I must make something perfectly clear. **Anyone who is severely depressed or suicidal, or has a history of drug or alcohol abuse, must be treated by a competent professional. Self-treatment is not an option.**

Most people do not suffer from serious depression. Subsyndromal, mild, and moderate depression are infinitely more common. But the sad fact is, many people simply learn to live with depression, at great personal expense. Maybe admitting to feeling depressed is too hard or too risky—there is still a social stigma attached to it. Maybe medical treatment is too costly, or maybe prescription antidepressants seem too harsh, too severe a step. Maybe the side effects of these antidepressants have been just too much to bear, a complaint I hear time and time again. Even if someone seeks medical help, chances are he or she will never see a psychopharmacologist, a psychiatrist, or any other mental health specialist. As most of you know, the growing trend toward managed care has reduced access to specialists of any kind. Today, depression is treated most often by primary care physicians. Unfortunately, the treatment of depression is tricky; studies show that sixty percent of the time, a primary care physician misses its symptoms. Even if depression is recognized, it is often treated inadequately. Only ten percent of all patients are receiving the appropriate antidepressant medication at the appropriate dose. That needs repeating. Ninety percent of people who seek medical help for depression are not being treated adequately. If ever there was an argument for a safe, over-the-counter treatment, it is that. Because SAM-e is so safe and easy to use, its availability will improve the odds that people who need treatment will get it, whether they are working with a doctor or not. It is increasingly incumbent upon patients to become the managers of their own health care, and for primary care physicians to become specialists in depression. *Stop Depression Now* works toward both those ends, giving doctors and patients the tools they need to better treat depression.

Why SAM-e, Why Now?

Many of you are probably thinking, if SAM-e is so good, why haven't we heard about it before? And more important, why doesn't my doctor know about it? When it comes to recognizing natural substances, the United States often lags behind the rest of the world. Why?

Economics. In the United States, information on antidepressants—and all other drugs—is effectively controlled by the pharmaceutical houses. I'm not criticizing them; far from it. Given the fact that the federal government has slashed its budget for scientific research, pharmaceutical companies have been forced to pick up the slack and have done so quite well. As a result, giant corporations beholden to their shareholders now fund most of the studies that appear in scientific journals, and inundate physicians with information on their new products. Unless a product is being marketed by a pharmaceutical company, physicians and the public never hear about it. Profit is the engine that drives new drug research and development, and for that reason, natural substances are frequently overlooked. Since under U.S. law it is very difficult to patent a natural substance, there is little incentive for a pharmaceutical company to invest the hundreds of millions of dollars in the clinical trials a drug needs to be approved by the Food and Drug Administration. Without a strong patent, a company could never recoup its investment before a competitor steps in. There is another factor as work here as well. Until recently, the United States had highly restrictive laws regarding the sale and marketing of natural supplements.

The net result was that no one wanted to back these natural substances as drugs, nor could you sell them over the counter. For that reason, many products sold over the counter for decades in Europe were simply unavailable in the United States. But in 1994, Congress passed the Dietary Supplement Health and Education Act (DSHEA), which cut through miles of regulatory red tape. Under the new law, any product with a good safety record can be quickly brought to market. This has been a boon to consumers because it has vastly increased their access to effective, proven supplements. However, the law has created new problems. For one thing, retailers and manufacturers are restricted in the claims they can make for a product, and the language they are forced to use on their packaging is often confusing. Consumers, as a result, have a difficult time even finding out about a good treatment option. As you know, doctors are no better informed. Few have any knowledge of supplements, how to use them, or how to separate the good from the bad. One of the reasons we are writing this book is to let the public know about this dramatic new supplement and to provide consumers and physicians with the information they need to use SAM-e safely and effectively. Because there is so little quality control of supplements in general, in Chapter 6 ("How to Take SAM-e") we are going to tell you what to look for when you buy SAM-e to ensure that you are getting the best, safest, and most effective product.

The Science of SAM-e: Two Decades of Research

Before you can fully understand why Terry and I are so excited about SAM-e, you need some background information. My father was in the U.S. military, and as a result, I spent a great deal of my childhood in Europe. Living in Europe taught me to appreciate different cultures, and I believe it made me more open-minded about many things. In fact, it introduced me to natural supplements, many of which were first developed in Europe, where they are sold side by side with conventional drugs. As a child I had two passions: spending time outdoors and studying chemistry. In college, I combined those interests by studying the chemistry of plants, a field which, unbeknownst to me, down the road would help me better understand natural medicine.

I began my medical studies in the mid-1970s, when the practice of psychiatry was undergoing a major transformation. Until the 1950s, psychoanalysis, the so-called "talking cure," was the primary treatment for depression. While there are many different schools of psychoanalysis, generally proponents of this form of treatment believe that depression is caused by life experience, whether an unconscious memory deeply buried or an image that can be vividly recalled. They believe that the only way to truly cure depression is to get to the root of the problem by enhancing self-understanding. Biology did not enter into the picture. If psychoanalysis did not work, which was often the case for severely depressed patients, the only other option was electroconvulsive therapy—shock treatment—which was surprisingly effective, but not too pleasant. It was used only when absolutely necessary.

By the 1960s, new drugs were introduced for the treatment of anxiety, opening the door to viewing all mental disorders as biological problems. Proponents of the so-called "drug revolution" in psychiatry believed that if a pill could relieve symptoms of anxiety that months or even years of psychotherapy could not, then depression might also be rooted in biochemistry. Research focused on a group of chemicals in the brain called neurotransmitters. These chemical messengers allow brain cells to communicate with one another, making thought possible. Imbalances in these brain chemicals were—and are—thought to cause depression. Work got under way on how to manipulate a person's neurotransmitters. By the 1970s, there were two categories of antidepressants in use: monoamine oxidase inhibitors—MAO inhibitors—and the tricyclic antidepressants.

These early classes of drugs—both still in use—did rescue many people from severe depression, but the side effects were often intolerable. Beneficial or not, many people just could not take them. MAO inhibitors and tricyclics were difficult to administer—they had to be carefully dosed and monitored. MAO inhibitors interact badly with certain common foods (cheese and wine, for example) and can be fatal when taken with widely used medications. The tricyclics posed another problem: in modest doses, they can be toxic, not exactly the kind of drug you wanted to prescribe for someone with suicidal tendencies.

I first heard about SAM-e twenty years ago during my residency in psychiatry (before a fellowship in psychiatry and psychobiology) at New York Hospital, Cornell Medical Center. A colleague who had just returned from a meeting of the American College of Neuropsychopharmacology was excited about a new antidepressant that was being studied in Europe. "It's better than what we have, it works faster, it's nontoxic, and there are no side effects," he marveled.

Two years later I asked him what happened to that new antidepressant he had been so enthusiastic about. "Well, you know, there are problems finding a company to fund research into a natural substance, you know, you can't patent it . . ."

The story might have ended there, but fifteen years later I was reintroduced to SAM-e by a patient. By that time I had established my own practice and had developed the subspecialty of treating patients resistant to conventional drug therapy. My particular interest and skill—my calling, if you will—is in helping patients for whom all other medicine has failed or has been intolerable. Since those early days of the drug revolution, there are new and better drugs in our antidepressant arsenal. In the late 1980s, the selective serotonin reuptake inhibitors (SRIs such as Prozac and Zoloft among many others) were approved for use in depression. These SRIs were about as effective as the drugs that preceded them, but they were easier to dose and had less severe side effects.

We may have made great strides in the use of medication to treat depression, but even these new drugs are far from perfect. They do not work all the time, nor do they work for everyone. Sometimes they stop working altogether after a while. It may surprise you to learn that even today one third of the population will not respond to standard antidepressant therapy, and twenty to thirty percent drop out of antidepressant studies due to side effects. These patients may require trying several different drugs, sometimes in combination, and special dosing. For them, finding something that works often takes years of grueling, side-effect-filled effort. In rare cases, nothing works.

Those patients who could not be helped by conventional medicine inspired me to explore alternative therapies. Soon, I developed an expertise in using unconventional treatments, often with great success. Not all my patients were looking for alternatives because conventional medication did not work. Some did not like the idea of taking a prescription drug—often for years on end—for which the long-term health effects were still unknown. Others preferred to use only natural substances whenever possible. Still others had health problems, such as heart disease or a history of liver disease, in which conventional antidepressants could be dangerous. And many patients decided they couldn't take the side effects any longer, even on the SRIs. Moreover, my concern about giving drugs that were so toxic in high doses never left me. Very often, I learned about new treatments from my patients, many of whom are intelligent, aware people who believe in taking an active role in managing their own health, and a substantial number of whom are themselves doctors.

That was the case with the patient who in 1994 put a bottle of SAM-e on my desk and a ream of material that she had gathered off the Internet. "I want to try this stuff," she said, "but only if you say it's okay."

I remembered SAM-e from my days as an intern, and her prodding was all I needed to begin to do research on the past fifteen years of use. I was very impressed by what I learned.

SUPERB RESEARCH. Since 1978, dozens of studies published in world-class scientific journals confirmed that SAM-e was a safe and effective antidepressant. It is nontoxic even at high doses.

AS GOOD AS OR BETTER THAN OTHER DRUGS. When tested against some of the most commonly used and most powerful antidepressants, patients showed a greater improvement on SAM-e in a shorter period of time. In one review article which analyzed more than a dozen clinical trials evaluating over a thousand patients taking SAM-e, the antidepressant response rate ranged from seventeen to thirty-eight percent better than those taking a placebo. To understand just how good this is, consider that standard antidepressants generally show an average response rate of about twenty percent over placebo.

NO SIDE EFFECTS, NO TOXICITY, NO WITHDRAWAL. Study after study showed me something particularly intriguing: SAM-e had a nearly total lack of side effects. Patients had more complaints about the sugar pill placebos than they did about SAM-e! Typically, in clinical studies of antidepressants, up to thirty percent of patients drop out because they cannot tolerate the side effects of the drug. Almost no one dropped out of the SAM-e studies. Moreover, SAM-e is completely nontoxic, even in very high doses. As an additional benefit, unlike other antidepressants SAM-e has no withdrawal period. To me, all this gave SAM-e a decided advantage over other antidepressants.

FASTER RESPONSE. Typically, it takes other antidepressants between four to six weeks to work. With SAM-e, patients usually showed improvement within a matter of days.

Despite the fact that current treatments are effective in managing depression, they are hardly panaceas. As noted earlier, it can take weeks or even months for patients to feel better. In the meantime, many actually feel worse, a whole lot worse. They get all the side effects of the medication with nothing to show for it. On top of their depression, they must now endure extremely unpleasant symptoms including dry mouth, headache, poor concentration, constipation, bladder problems, nausea, and the two that patients complain about the most—weight gain and sexual dysfunction. We doctors often cavalierly dismiss these patients as neurotic, uncooperative, or ungrateful, and there have been articles in medical journals devoted to the personality flaws of patients who refuse to stay on their antidepressants. Why, we wonder, don't they want to get well? Recently, one of my colleagues, a highly esteemed psychiatrist, admitted that he used to think there was something inherently wrong with patients who refused to stay on antidepressants. A champion of SRIs, he believed that because these drugs were so easy to dose—and therefore so easy for doctors to use—they were *the* answer to depression. That was until he started taking Prozac himself. After two weeks, he was so unhappy with the side effects (inhibition of orgasm was the one that bothered him most) that he discontinued it and tried a different type of antidepressant. On that drug, he got dry mouth, and this sharp, highly intelligent, well-focused man felt spacey. He couldn't stay on either drug long enough to see his depression lift. He's changed his mind about prescription antidepressants. "Unless you've tried the damn medication you don't know how bad it is," he says. (Now he uses

SAM-e, his depression is gone, and so are the side effects.)

I also learned how SAM-e was being used in Europe to treat a number of different illnesses unrelated to depression. Since safety is a primary concern in medicine, I was relieved to read a particular study that showed that SAM-e had been used successfully to treat a liver problem that occurs late in pregnancy. Women had been given high doses of SAM-e for up to twenty days to treat intrahepatic cholestasis (obstruction of the bile tract). It did not cause any problems with the pregnancy or harm the baby in any way. Numerous other safety studies told similar tales.

Convinced of both its safety and efficacy, I began to incorporate SAM-e into my practice. I had great success. Since 1994, I have prescribed SAM-e to hundreds of patients, many of whom have had major drug-resistant depression. If a patient suffers from mild-to-moderate depression, often the first thing I try is SAM-e. Typically, within a week of starting it, many patients report dramatic improvement in their symptoms. In cases of severe depression, patients may need higher doses of SAM-e than I ordinarily recommend, or need to take it in combination with another medication. I will tell you more about how to use SAM-e in Chapter 6 ("How to Take SAM-e").

A word of warning: **If you are taking a prescription antidepressant, do not discontinue it abruptly and start on SAM-e. If you do, you could develop** withdrawal symptoms, which could be extremely unpleasant. Rather, you should work with your doctor to cut back gradually on your prescription antidepressant—in the hopes of eliminating it entirely—while taking SAM-e. (See Chapter 6 for more details.)

Depression Has Been Neglected

Like other mental disorders, depression is not perceived to be life-threatening, as is cancer or heart disease, and thus has been neglected and marginalized by the public. Mental disorders still have a stigma, a badge of shame about them that we don't hang on other health problems. No one sponsors a walkathon to help fund research on depression; no one shows up at the Academy Awards wearing a colored ribbon to remind people that depression is a serious health hazard. But it's every bit as serious and even more widespread than the common illnesses that do get all the attention. There is a fifteen percent suicide rate among the seriously depressed; that is a high mortality rate for any disease. Unhealthy behaviors such as smoking, drug abuse, and alcohol abuse may also be linked to depression.

Depression is costly in other ways as well. The economic burden of depression in the United States is $43.7 billion a year, with only $12 billion of that in direct costs for physician visits, hospital stays, and medication (which itself accounts for only three percent of the total cost). The indirect costs of depression are staggering. Depression causes more days in bed—and absences from work—than diabetes, arthritis, lung problems, and gastrointestinal problems *combined*. According to the World Health Organization, depression accounts for five percent of the global burden for disease, placing it ahead of heart disease and cancer. Only infectious diseases and malnutrition afflict more people. The personal cost of depression is equally high. It can not only destroy an individual's life but also damage an entire family. In addition, it increases the risk of developing other serious illnesses, such as heart disease and dementia, down the road. Depression is also a recurrent, even chronic, disease—once you've been depressed, you have a very high risk of becoming depressed again.

Those who suffer from depression are often reluctant to admit it. People who are unaware of the true nature of depression may dismiss it as a sign of weakness, a character flaw, or even just a lousy personality. With that kind of reception awaiting them, many find it difficult to step forward and get the help they need. In addition, they may not want to get help, particularly if their health insurance is provided by their employer. Many sufferers, probably wisely, do not want their employers to know they have a problem with depression. In other cases, they are afraid—and rightfully so—that they will be discriminated against if they seek treatment. Recently, several of my patients were turned down for long-term disability insurance because the insurance carrier learned they were taking prescription antidepressants. (As noted above, depression increases the risk of developing other medical problems, a fact that is considered in actuarial tables.) Having been labeled bad risks, they were refused insurance. By the way, I believe that treating depression in a timely fashion may greatly reduce the odds of developing long-term health problems. But insurance companies, not known for their flexibility, do not take this into account.

One of the reasons why SAM-e holds such promise as a treatment for depression is that people can obtain it for themselves easily, quietly, and privately. Hopefully, many people who would not have sought treatment otherwise will now find relief—faster than they ever thought possible. There is absolutely no question that SAM-e is safe; in fact, as I have mentioned and will discuss later, it offers some intriguing health benefits.

About ninety percent of people with depression have what is known as unipolar depression— that is, characterized by a down mood. The remainder are bipolar, also known as manic-depressive; they swing from periods of intense sadness to periods of manic highs. These people should not use SAM-e or any other antidepressant except under a doctor's supervision, since it can shift them into a manic period.

The Side Benefits of SAM-e

When I prescribe medication on a regular basis for my patients, I can't help worrying about the long-term health effects of those drugs. Frankly, we don't know the effect of taking Prozac, Zoloft, or Wellbutrin for twenty or thirty years or beyond. It's never been studied, and the drugs haven't been around long enough to see what happens to long-term users. But we do know that depression itself is life-threatening, and therefore there is no doubt in my mind that these medications are essential. When I prescribe SAM-e, however, I don't have any of these concerns. Both Terry and I believe that it is not only powerful medicine against depression, but is health-enhancing in many other ways.

When I first began researching SAM-e, I was astounded by the number of studies that had been performed on this little-known molecule. It became apparent that even though physicians like myself were unaware of SAM-e, it was the subject of intense study by biochemists like Terry. I wondered, why was SAM-e attracting so much scientific attention?

From a biochemist's point of view, SAM-e is as good as it gets. It is a molecule that lies at the crossroads of a multitude of important biochemical reactions in the body. It is vital for life. A critical component of the chemical process called methylation, SAM-e is involved in nearly every activity in the body, from growth and development to protecting us against disease.

How to Use this Book

The Stop Depression Now program consists of four simple steps, each one designed to lift you out of depression and prevent a recurrence. I often describe this program as a four-legged chair. Remove or weaken one leg—no matter which one—and it becomes unstable, prone to tipping you off balance and back onto the floor. No one leg is more or less important than the others. It is important to follow each of these steps to get good results.

Step 1 • **ASSESS YOUR MOOD.** The first step on the road to beating depression is finding out where you are now. That is why we've included a simple but widely respected self-test. This is an adaptation of the self-evaluation that many psychiatrists and psychologists administer to their patients to evaluate depression. It is an essential tool for figuring out whether you have subsyndromal, mild, moderate, or even severe depression. (**Remember: If you suffer from severe depression, this book is no substitute for professional psychiatric help. Please see your doctor.**) Your score on this self-test will allow you to find the right SAM-e dose for you. By periodically reevaluating yourself, you can see how well you are progressing.

Step 2 • **TAKE SAM-E.** Now it is time to deal with the biochemical imbalance that may be at the root of your depression. Chapter 6 ("How to Take SAM-e") will tell you exactly how much SAM-e you need, how to take it, and when you can expect to start feeling better. (It's surprisingly fast!) You will also learn what kind of SAM-e to buy—and what kind to avoid.

Step 3 • **EAT THE RIGHT FOOD.** Our modern diet may be a contributing factor to the high incidence of depression. Step 3, as outlined in Chapter 7 ("The Stop Depression Now Food Plan"), deals with the link between nutrition and mental health. Here you will find essential information on what foods can make you feel better and what ones can leave you blue. You will discover what vitamins and minerals make your SAM-e work even better and how to make your body help fight depression.

Step 4 • **ADOPT THE RIGHT LIFESTYLE.** Following Steps 1, 2, and 3 will lift you out of your depression and make you feel a lot better. But in order to *stay* depression-free, you will probably need to make some constructive changes in your lifestyle. Chapter 8 ("A Simple Guide to Depression-Proofing Your Life"), will introduce you to cutting-edge cognitive therapy you can use on yourself, and to tried-and-true techniques patients have been using for years to stay depression-free.

One of the first steps in treating your depression is understanding what depression is all about, and recognizing the enormous impact it has on your life and the lives of your loved ones. In Chapter 2 ("What Is Depression?") I will discuss the latest scientific information on the causes of depression, and explain why getting prompt and effective treatment is so important.

2

What Is Depression?

"I was chronically depressed for nearly all of my life. I didn't get any pleasure out of living—I couldn't really enjoy anything. Any happiness was temporary, very fleeting, and then I would go right back into the dumps. I didn't expect SAM-e to work, I had been through so many other medications including St. John's wort. Nothing worked well. With SAM-e I've had a big response. I've never felt better in my life. I get much more pleasure out of life. I'm much more active, I'm much more resilient. I still get down . . . but I'm better able to cope."

M.K.

"I never had a bout of severe depression, but every few months or so I would have some very, very bad days. It would just come and go, and it went on for years. I tried several other an-

tidepressants, but I couldn't stay on them because I hated the side effects. Since I've been taking SAM-e, I haven't had any of those low days. I've been feeling consistently pretty good."

L.P.

Both of these patients suffer from depression, yet their experiences are remarkably different. The first has endured a lifetime of severe depression. Now that he is taking SAM-e, he has found relief for the first time in his life. He is no longer stuck in the emotional wasteland that has plagued him since childhood. The other patient wrestles with a milder form of depression—brief yet recurrent episodes of feeling blue. Although on the surface he is able to function well in the world, it is not without personal struggle. He never knew when the dark days would strike. Now that he too is taking SAM-e, he no longer lives under a cloud.

Nearly everyone has experienced feelings of depression—feeling down or blue is an essential part of the normal range of human emotion. In life, things happen that can make us profoundly sad—sometimes for days, weeks, or even months at a time. In fact, many would say that without an occasional sad mood, you would be unable to fully appreciate the joyous moments of life! I heartily agree. Sad moments are rich, valuable, and a key component of a full life. The point of *Stop Depression Now* is not that you should *never* experience a depressed feeling, but rather to keep you from spending your life languishing in sadness and despair.

There is a real difference between being in a bad mood—or even being quite sad, down, or blue—and being depressed. A nondepressed person can usually shake off a bad mood on his or her own. That is utter fantasy for someone in the grip of depression. Depression is a chronic, often debilitating problem that sabotages your ability to heal yourself. It is not something you can just "snap out of" or "get over." It interferes with your life in countless ways, from damaging your intimate relationships to alienating your friends, from making work a misery to hurting your future prospects. Even worse, depression is hazardous to your health. Be it in the form of heart disease or cancer, suppressed immunity or weight gain, depression is—literally—a killer. And you are not the only one that your depression is hurting. Depressed parents often lack the resilience or patience to fully nurture their children, even neglecting them emotionally or physically. Is it any wonder that depression passes from one generation to the next? Depression is no less brutal on your friends and family. For people who care for you, there is no worse feeling than watching you hurt—especially when there is nothing, it seems, that can be done. In the worst cases, depression can even drive off those on whom you love and depend. At the very least, depression casts a gray pall over everything, preventing you from enjoying the good things in life. In its most severe form, it can make life seem not worth living.

There Is Hope

"I am now the most miserable man living. If what I feel were equally distributed to the whole human family, there would be not one cheerful face on earth. Whether I shall be better, I cannot tell . . . To remain as I am is impossible. I must die or be better, it appears to me."

When Abraham Lincoln uttered those words of despair, there was little that could be done about what he called the "melancholia" that afflicted him for most of his life. People had no choice but to simply live with depression regardless of the impact it had on their lives. If depression became so serious that you could no longer function in society, you were often confined to your home or even locked away in an asylum. It is no coincidence that gothic novels are replete with tales of "insane" relatives who were hidden away in the attic of the family home. This scenario was not just born from the vivid imagination of Victorian authors—it was a reality of nineteenth-century life. In all likelihood, many people back then who were diagnosed as insane were, in fact, psychotically depressed—that is, so severely ill that they would actually develop symptoms like hallucinations and delusions. While no one need suffer like that today—especially with the advent of SAM-e—in those days there was little to offer. The picture of depression treatment has changed dramatically over the last century, and Terry and I believe it's about to change again, once more for the better.

The first step in dealing with depression is acknowledging that you are depressed. This chapter will explain what depression is, how to recognize it, and ultimately how to shed it. It will also help you to better understand what depression is all about.

You're Not Alone

Depression has been called the "common cold" of psychiatric ailments. It is epidemic in modern society. As noted in Chapter 1, it is the number one complaint that primary care doctors are called upon to diagnose and treat. More widespread than diabetes, heart disease, and even cancer, major depression afflicts more than 17 million Americans each year. Countless others suffer from milder forms and undiagnosed cases of depression. It may surprise you—and unsettle you—to learn that you have a thirty percent risk of developing a serious adult depression over the course of your life. If we consider the other forms of milder depression, that risk rises to about fifty percent. Fifty percent! That means *one person in two* will find him- or herself depressed at some point in life.

But your risk of depression varies depending on your age and gender, and even where you live. Women are twice as likely to be diagnosed with depression as men. However, I believe the rate of depression among men is almost certainly underreported, because men do not seek medical attention as readily as women. Depression among the elderly, often overlooked as well, is two to three times more common than among the young. In fact, the rate of *serious* depression in nursing homes and hospitals could be as high as twenty percent. It is very easy to dismiss depression among the elderly as dementia or even a natural consequence of aging, but it's not. It's depression all the same, and no one should have to endure it because he or she is old. That's just plain cruel. It should be treated as vigorously as depression among any other age group. (See Chapter 11, "Getting Healthy With SAM-e.")

There are several types of depression that affect people at different times of their lives, and even different times of the year:

SEASONAL AFFECTIVE DISORDER. Some people—especially those who live in the Northeast and Upper Midwest—may get depressed only during the fall and winter months. For some, it can begin as early as the end of September and last until May. When sunshine is scarce these folks feel blue. Called seasonal affective disorder, or SAD, this condition has only recently been recognized by mainstream medicine, and it is still controversial. People with SAD feel sluggish and lethargic, often overeating and oversleeping during the fall and winter. They may get weepy and morose. Very often, their performance at school or on the job declines during the sun-deprived months and peaks during the spring and summer. As one patient who suffers from SAD describes it, "In the fall, when the light changes, I would feel claustrophobic, like the darkness was closing in on me. I felt like I was smothered by a blanket of despair. It's a horrible, horrible feeling." Fortunately, a combination of SAM-e and light therapy has brought her out of the darkness.

POSTPARTUM DEPRESSION. From fifty to eighty percent of all new mothers experience some postpartum blues—mood swings and crying—which usually go away within ten days of giving birth. It's understandable that women would feel down after having a baby. For one thing, caring for a newborn is exhausting. For another, it can take up to several weeks for the body's hormonal balance to return to normal, which could contribute to chemical imbalances that cause mood swings. Up to fifteen percent of new mothers, however, suffer from a more serious form of postpartum blues that looks and feels like clinical depression. For information on how SAM-e can help, read Chapter 9 ("Good News for Women"). Note: **A sizable percentage of women with postpartum depression are in the bipolar spectrum. These women may develop hypomania on SAM-e.**

POSTMENOPAUSAL DEPRESSION. The postmenopausal years are a vulnerable time for women, especially those who are depression-prone. Similar to postpartum depression, postmenopausal depression may be linked to specific hormonal changes brought about by the decline in estrogen and other key hormones. Midlife is also a time of change in many women's lives. Children leave home, parents get sick and die, careers may be in transition and lifestyles in flux. All of these changes—good or bad—can be stressful and can contribute to depression.

DEPRESSION OF CHRONIC ILLNESS. Depression is a common problem among people who are chronically ill, but it is often neglected. When people have life-threatening or debilitating ailments such as heart disease, cancer, or diabetes, the focus is on maintaining their physical health. If they are depressed, it is often dismissed as par for the course. Unfortunately, depression can hamper the body's ability to heal and repair itself, further aggravating an already bad situation. (The good news is that because of its lack of side effects—and its overall health benefits—SAM-e is a good choice for people who are suffering from the depression of chronic illness.

Depression: Getting to a Diagnosis

Despite the fact that depression is so widespread, it is still underdiagnosed, undertreated, and often misunderstood . . . even by doctors. As we discussed in the last chapter, depression still carries a social stigma. We like to think of ourselves as enlightened—no longer do we lock our depressed relatives away in the attic—yet when it comes to recognizing mental illness, we are still very much in the dark. People who have not had experience with depression may mistakenly believe that it is a voluntary condition; if *they* can rise above a bad mood, the blues, or a setback, then why can't everybody else? The depressed person gets blamed for not trying hard enough. He or she is accused of seeking attention, having a character flaw, or being weak-willed. I'm sure many of you have been told by friends and relatives that you were wallowing in your unhappiness and you could snap out of it if you really wanted to. What these well-meaning friends and relatives don't realize is that depression is not some illusory behavioral problem—it is the result of biochemical changes that disrupt the body and the brain's biology. To treat depression effectively, that biochemical imbalance must be corrected in addition to helping people learn better coping skills.

In recent years, in order to destigmatize depression, it has become popular to refer to it as an illness. On one hand, this is good because it reminds us that, as with other ailments like heart disease or cancer, people who are depressed don't have a choice. They are not being difficult or obstinate—their problems are very real and as biological as any other illness. On the other hand, however, it artificially separates those who are depressed from those who are not. Granted, there may be people who are more emotionally resilient than others due to good genetics or good parenting or a combination of both. But if confronted with a horrible enough set of events, even the most resilient among us could become clinically depressed. We are learning that brain chemistry can be powerfully influenced by circumstance, so that while events may bring on depression, its manifestation is chemical. And no one is immune. *No one.* That is one reason why I prefer to call depression a vulnerability rather than an illness. Furthermore, an illness implies symptoms but a vulnerability does not.

It is often difficult to diagnose depression, especially for primary care doctors who are not necessarily experts in the field. Unlike medical conditions such as high blood pressure or high cholesterol levels, there is no quick and easy test that will lead a doctor to a diagnosis of depression. The tools of modern medicine—expensive machines, blood tests, and the like—are strangely silent on the subject. Unless the depression is severe and obvious, recognizing it may require spending time talking to the patient—something that has been lost in the "medicine by stopwatch" atmosphere of managed care. Often, the depressed person him- or herself may have to step forward and ask for help, and ironically, the more depressed the person is, the less likely he or she is to acknowledge it. Severely depressed patients will sooner believe that they are physically ill or even dying than accept that they are depressed. Or they will blame their problems on other people—"My husband hates me," "It's all my boss's fault"—blind to the true cause of their suffering. It is one of depression's cruel tricks. Very often, it is a concerned parent or spouse who insists that they get help.

To further complicate the problem, a depressed person may complain of a litany of physical ailments, such as insomnia, chronic pain, or fatigue, every one of them real and often brought on by the depression itself. It's no wonder primary care doctors have trouble sorting out the true problem.

Sometimes the opposite is the case. Depression may be a symptom of another underlying medical problem that may be overlooked in the haste to diagnose. Studies show that forty percent of patients admitted to psychiatric hospitals for depression have a physical ailment that has either caused or aggravated their depression. Just as depression can be overlooked, so can other conditions be confused with depression. All too often, doctors and patients confuse complaints like fatigue or irritability with depression when in fact they are caused by hormonal disorders, nutritional deficiencies, autoimmune diseases, heart disease, cancer, or even substance abuse. That is why I recommend that everyone who feels depressed (or has been diagnosed with depression) undergo a thorough physical examination.

If depression accompanies another condition and you fix the underlying problem, the depression doesn't magically go away. It still must be treated. This point is particularly important for mildly depressed people who may want to take SAM-e without consulting with their doctor. Unless you have had a thorough physical examination (which is something every adult should do on an annual basis), I don't recommend that you take SAM-e. I'm not worried about the safety of SAM-e—in fact, it will probably help you—but I *am* worried that you won't get proper medical treatment if you do have an underlying problem.

To give you an idea of how closely linked physical illness and depression are, here is a list of ailments and medications that can cause depression:

SOME MEDICAL CONDITIONS AND TREATMENTS THAT CAN CAUSE, MIMIC, OR AGGRAVATE DEPRESSION

Autoimmune Diseases • Lyme disease, viral hepatitis, viral meningitis, encephalitis, pneumonia, HIV, mononucleosis, influenza, tuberculosis

Brain Diseases • Post stroke, Parkinson's, Alzheimer's, vascular dementia, traumatic brain injury, multiple sclerosis, Huntington's, Wilson's, Lewy body disease, temporal lobe epilepsy, subdural hematoma

Dietary Deficiences • Deficiencies of B_6, B_{12}, folate, or thiamine; scurvy (caused by a severe deficiency in vitamin C)

Heart Disease • Mitral valve prolapse and congestive heart failure

Metabolic • Kidney disease, mineral imbalances (especially potassium, sodium, and calcium)

TREATMENTS

Heart Disease • Beta blockers, reserpine, methyldopa, clonidine, calcium channel blockers, digoxin, anti-arrhythmics, cholesterol-reducing drugs, cardiac surgery, and immunosuppressive drugs after transplant surgery

Lung Disease • Corticosteroids

Cancer • Many chemotherapy agents, steroids, interferon

Infection • Cycloserine, isonazid, acyclovir, ciproflaxacin, mefloquine

Brain Disorders • Levodopa, dopamine agonists, anticonvulsants, painkillers

Skin Disorders • Isotretinoin, Dapsone

Gastrointestinal Disorders • Metoclopramide, histamine receptor blockers, non-steroidal anti-inflammatory drugs (NSAIDs)

Depression Is a Chronic Health Problem

One of the primary reasons to diagnose and treat depression properly is that if you don't, it will almost always recur, for reasons that I will explain later. In fact, if untreated, the rate of recurrence of a first episode of severe depression is as high as fifty percent. Even if it is treated, with every severe depressive episode the risk of recurrence rises substantially. It is critical to diagnose and treat depression as early as possible. Keep in mind that an untreated mild depression can rapidly turn into a more severe problem. The more severe the depression, the more difficult it is to treat and the more vulnerable you may be to recurrence down the road. Therefore, it is important to be able to identify the early stages of depression so that you can intervene quickly and effectively. Proper treatment often halts the downward spiral and begins the healing process. Because SAM-e works so quickly and effectively, it can accelerate the rate of recovery, reducing the risk of a mild depression spiraling out of control.

The Signs of Depression

As we have seen, there are two categories of depression—unipolar and bipolar (also known as manic depression). The overwhelming majority of people—

about ninety-five percent—suffer from unipolar depression. People with unipolar depression feel low, sad, and slowed down. On the other hand, those with bipolar depression are thrown into the roller coaster of periods of severe depression alternating with high-energy, manic periods that seem out of touch with reality. As noted earlier, this book is written for those with unipolar depression. Those with bipolar depression need to be under the care and treatment of a physician, particularly since all standard antidepressants—even the herb St. John's wort—may aggravate their problem and send them into a manic episode.

For most people, the word "depression" is synonymous with sadness or feeling blue, but sadness is just one of the many signs of depression, and there are even more significant symptoms. Although depression may be experienced by different people in profoundly different ways, I have listed its most common signs below.

FEELING EMPTY OR FLAT. One of the most common complaints I hear from my depressed patients is of feeling "empty" or "flat" to the point that they are unable to get any enjoyment out of life. They don't experience the normal range of emotion—they are stuck in neutral, looking out over a featureless emotional landscape.

INNER FEELINGS OF SADNESS. Not surprisingly, feeling blue or down is a typical symptom of depression. Happy occasions do not elevate the spirits of depressed people; they may even make them feel worse. On the other hand, sad occasions may send them into a downward spiral of hopelessness.

LOCKED IN NEGATIVE FEELINGS. People with depression live in a world where their past, present, and future look bleak. Things, they believe, will only get worse. Positive thoughts drown in a flood of negativity.

FEELING TENSE AND NERVOUS. It may come as a surprise to you that being nervous and high-strung is a very common sign of depression. Depressed people may fidget a great deal and seem to be on edge. They'll pull on their hair or clothes, tear apart paper or shred a Styrofoam cup, and often appear agitated.

LOSS OF INTEREST IN LIFE. Depression and apathy often go hand in hand. Unable to muster up interest in daily activities, depressed people detach, becoming socially isolated, lonely, and mired in low-level, running boredom. The spouses and significant others of depressed people say that their partners are no longer engaging in activities they once enjoyed, including sex, or even participating in family life.

FEELING GUILTY AND WORTHLESS. Depressed people tend to blame themselves for everything. They will think (and sometimes say), "I'm a total failure. I can't stand myself. My wife should leave me. I blame myself for everything bad that happens." Their own worst enemies, they systematically destroy their self-esteem. For this reason, telling a depressed person to "shape up" can do further damage. They can't just snap out of it, and now they have a new reason to think of themselves as failures—too inadequate to even control their own moods.

DIFFICULTY CONCENTRATING AND MAKING DECISIONS. Depression often robs you of your ability to focus and perform simple mental tasks. Very often, depressed people have difficulty making clear decisions. Depression clouds the brain and leaves its sufferers unfocused. Obviously, this can have disastrous consequences at school or work or in relationships with others. In some cases, depression can lead to memory problems.

SLEEP PROBLEMS. If you find yourself waking up earlier than usual in the morning and being unable to fall back to sleep, you may be experiencing one of the early signs of depression. In more severe depressions, people may have problems falling asleep and may wake up several times during the night. No wonder many depressed people walk around feeling absolutely exhausted! Sleep deprivation could also explain why depression leads to the cognitive problems described above.

CHANGE IN APPETITE. Typically, a depressed person begins to lose weight. He or she is not eating as much as usual and doesn't seem to care about food. This is often a reflection of the fact that when you are depressed you stop taking care of yourself, and nothing is more basic to self-care than nourishment.

Making matters worse, a poor diet and nutritional deficiencies can aggravate depression. In some cases, depression can trigger overeating and weight gain. Some people use food to elevate their mood, and depression brings on eating binges they would never have given in to before. A sudden change in appetite or weight is a common sign of a problem.

CHANGE IN ACTIVITY LEVEL. Depressed people may seem slow and sluggish and have trouble dragging themselves out of bed. In some cases, however, their activity level can speed up. As with appetite, any sudden change in activity level in combination with these other symptoms could indicate depression.

SUICIDAL THOUGHTS. When life is giving you nothing but misery, death seems like the most attractive solution. Talk of suicide or suicidal actions should never be dismissed—there is a fifteen percent suicide rate among the severely depressed. There should be no mistake about this: **People who are severely depressed or suicidal must be under a doctor's supervision. It is not up to a friend or relative to decide whether or not they are really serious about killing themselves. If you or someone you know is suicidal—or even if you just suspect it—*get professional help.* Severe depression has a higher mortality rate than heart disease!** It is not uncommon, however, for even people with milder depression to feel on occasion that life's not worth living or to have fleeting suicidal thoughts. They may wish to be put out of their misery by having a heart attack or being run over by a car, but they are not necessarily going to actively take their own life. Once again, it's a matter of degree. If you have any suicidal thoughts— recurrent, occasional, whatever—you must get professional help.

Some of you may have experienced most or all of these signs of depression, while others may identify with only one or two. Some may feel these emotions acutely, while others may have such thoughts and feelings intermittently. The fact is, *feelings of depression are universal.* The difference is in the degree to which they are felt. That is why in Chapter 6 ("How to Take SAM-e") you'll find a self-test—one used by professionals—that helps you rate your depression based on the severity of your symptoms. The results of this test will allow you to personalize your treatment program while giving you a tool to periodically evaluate your progress.

In general, doctors characterize patients exhibiting the worst symptoms for at least two weeks as having severe depression which should be treated. Those with fewer or less intense symptoms are diagnosed with moderate depression. Dysthymia signifies milder depression over a two-year period or longer; this may or may not interfere with your ability to perform life's functions, but it will certainly hamper your ability to enjoy life. Some psychiatrists, myself included, are beginning to believe that there are countless other people walking around with very low, but very real, levels of depression. As noted in Chapter 1, this subsyndromal depression or intermittent minor depression can best be described as feeling down or blue. At one time, we dismissed these mild depressions as character flaws and placed them in a separate category from true chemical depressions. Now there is a growing realization that low-level depressions may also be caused by mildly abnormal biochemistry.

There is still a great deal of controversy as to whether these low-level mood disorders are true depressions that require treatment. It is one of the gray zones of psychiatry, areas in which there are few hard-and-fast rules and even less agreement among professionals.

The longer I practice medicine, however, the more I realize that these labels and distinctions are often arbitrary and artificial. Depression is ultimately a subjective experience. Some people can go on for years with the same set of symptoms that would send someone else running to the doctor for help.

It is for this very reason that SAM-e is of such benefit. It can be a great help not only to those with standard severe or mild-to-moderate depressions, but also to those of you who may be stuck in the gray zone of subsyndromal depression. Even if you've hesitated to see a doctor for whatever reason, SAM-e's safety and easy availability will, I'm sure, help countless numbers of you who would not otherwise be helped. SAM-e is no less a blessing for those who have been reluctant to use other antidepressants because of their side effects or concerns about their impact on long-term health. The benefits are no less clear for people currently taking prescription antidepressants and finding them almost as intolerable as the depression itself.

What Causes Depression?

Identifying depression is the easy part; getting to its root cause has proven far more difficult. Although we have discovered a great deal about the biology of depression within the past few decades, there is still much more to learn. We have but a few pieces in what will undoubtedly turn out to be a complex puzzle, larger than we can imagine from our current vantage point. Debate still rages over the extent to which depression is a biological event versus one that is rooted in past experiences and present environment. These issues may continue to be hotly debated, but there is a growing patch of common ground.

Here's what scientists do agree upon. Depression stems from a combination of chemical imbalances and environmental factors. Some people may be born with a particular biochemical vulnerability that can result in depression under the right circumstances. Others who are not necessarily born with a vulnerability may have life experiences that can just as readily trigger depression. It is not easy to distinguish between a depression caused by a biochemical glitch and a depression caused by a life event. Of course, to the depressed person, it all feels very much the same.

In order to better understand depression, you need to know a bit about how the brain works. Weighing less than two pounds, the human brain is nature's greatest marvel and one of the hardest-working organs in the body. The repository of reasoning, intellect, memory, consciousness, and emotion, the brain also coordinates all of the body's activities. It controls not only those activities that we do voluntarily, like picking up the phone, walking across the room, or reading a book, but also those that we do unconsciously like our heartbeat, breathing, and digestion. In order to do all this hard work, the brain consists of billions of specialized cells called neurons. Neurons "talk" with each other via a vast network of tiny branchlike connections called dendrites. These dendrites may form a tangled web, but they do not actually touch one another. There are trillions of tiny gaps between them, called synapses. Nerve impulses—chemical messages—travel from one neuron to the other by releasing chemicals called neurotransmitters which move from the dendrite across the synapse to another dendrite. The neurotransmitter then binds to a receptor on the dendrite, triggering an electrochemical response in the attached neuron which causes the release of more neurotransmitters. Once they are used, neurotransmitters are either "recycled"—that is, taken back up by the neuron to be used again—or eliminated from the body by being sent from the brain to the cerebrospinal fluid, and from there into the bloodstream, and eventually passed as urine. How well the body recycles the neurotransmitters it needs, and disposes of those it doesn't, is critical in the depression story.

There are literally tens of millions of these dendrite-neuron-synapse-dendrite-neuron connections being made at any one time. Think about it. Every time you breathe, walk, talk, blink an eye, or even smile, millions of brain cells are involved in coordinating the activity. Neurotransmitters are the oil that keeps the brain and the body running smoothly—they are absolutely vital for normal brain function. And maintaining the right balance between them is key to a well-functioning person. Since the 1960s, researchers have suspected that a decline in one or more key neurotransmitters may somehow cause depression. Research has focused on three particular neurotransmitters, the monoamines: noradrenaline (also known as norepinephrine,) serotonin, and dopamine. Noradrenaline is involved in our response to stress and anxiety. Serotonin is instrumental in many different activities, including the regulation of hormones, appetite control, sexual behavior, and sleeping. Dopamine helps control physical movement, and an imbalance in dopamine may also cause a loss of reality that can result in hallucinations and delusions. In fact, such an imbalance is believed to be a factor in schizophrenia.

Depressed patients may have lower-than-normal levels of monoamines in their spinal fluid, which suggests that there are lower levels of these chemicals in their brains. But how these monoamines are involved in depression has remained a subject of debate.

Initially, researchers wavered between believing the real problem was too much noradrenaline or too little, but they later settled on an imbalance between noradrenaline and the other neurotransmitters. Two important classes of antidepressants, the MAO inhibitors and the tricyclics, both work by helping the brain maintain normal noradrenaline levels. MAO inhibitors are so named because they block the action of an enzyme (monoamine oxidase), which therefore boosts monoamine levels. As a result, the neuron has more of the precious neurotransmitter to reuse. In a different way, tricyclic antidepressants also prevent the loss of noradrenaline. (For a more complete description of antidepressants, see Chapter 4, "The Antidepressant Arsenal.")

In the 1980s, researchers turned their focus to serotonin, after low levels of serotonin had been linked to suicide. Their efforts produced a class of highly effective drugs (such as Prozac) known as the serotonin reuptake inhibitors, or SRIs, which did for serotonin what the MAO inhibitors and tricyclics did for noradrenaline. As you may have gathered by now, depression can stem from a problem with any of the neurotransmitters. Finding the right treatment for depression depends on finding the particular system afflicted, a hit-or-miss proposition to this day. What makes SAM-e unique among antidepressants is that it boosts levels of both serotonin and dopamine, while stabilizing noradrenaline levels, allowing for a much broader and faster effect.

Why is maintaining the balance between neurotransmitters so important? Once again, there are several plausible explanations. First, neurotransmitters may help the body and the mind better cope with stress, which can trigger depression in susceptible people. When we are under stress, our bodies produce a hormone called cortisol which, as I explain later, can be harmful, especially to our brain cells. Although the precise mechanism is not known, properly balanced neurotransmitters may prevent release of excess cortisol. Second, neurotransmitters may help regulate a sort of clock in the brain that controls the timing of events in the body. Like every other animal on the planet, human beings follow particular daily and seasonal rhythms which, if disrupted, can create both physical and emotional problems. Remember, one of the symptoms of depression is a change of activity, either a speeding up in the case of bipolar depression, or a slowing down as in the case of the more common unipolar depression. In addition, many of the other symptoms of depression, such as insomnia or change in appetite, are also related to the inability of the body to maintain a normal biological cycle. When you don't maintain a normal biological cycle, your body will not produce key hormones at the appropriate times or in the right amounts, which ultimately will disrupt the production of neurotransmitters. The bigger questions, of

course, are: What causes an imbalance in neurotransmitters in the first place, and why does it happen to
some people and not others? In some cases, the answer
lies in our genes. Certain people may be born with a
tendency to underproduce neurotransmitters. However, it's not a matter of genetics alone. Being born
with this genetic vulnerability doesn't necessarily mean
that you will get depressed. Nor does it mean that if
you are born without this vulnerability, you are immune.

Life isn't that simple, and that's the point. There
are many factors to consider, including life experience.
Childhood trauma can set the stage for adult depression. If, during childhood, you lose a parent to divorce,
illness, or death, the risk of developing depression as an
adult is very high, regardless of your genetic makeup.
If you live in a strife-ridden area like Beirut or Kosovo,
you are more likely to be depressed than if you live in
a calm, peaceful environment. Clearly, things can happen in our lives that can affect our body chemistry in
a profoundly negative way.

Stress As a Trigger for Depression

When I was in medical school, I was taught that there
was a difference between biological depression—the
kind caused by a biochemical imbalance—and depression caused by a traumatic event, such as a death or
similar loss. In fact, it was drilled into us that antide-

pressants were only useful for true biological depressions, and that so-called "event depressions" would heal spontaneously on their own. Current research challenges this point of view, and the lines between biological and event depressions are beginning to blur. The link between both types of depression is the body's response to stress.

Close your eyes and imagine yourself living back in the days of the caveman. You're out picking berries for breakfast and suddenly you're staring into the face of a saber-toothed tiger who is also foraging for food—you. He growls and bares his teeth. Understandably, you are terrified. Without any design on your part, your stress-response system swings into action. It is an instinctual response controlled by the autonomic (involuntary) nervous system, the same system that regulates other automatic reactions such as breathing or the beating of your heart. Your brain orders a series of physiological responses that gear the body up for action. Your adrenal glands begin to pump higher levels of stress hormones—adrenaline, noradrenaline, and cortisol—into your bloodstream. Your kidneys release another hormone, renin, which raises blood pressure and forces the heart to pump faster. Blood is diverted from your stomach toward your skeletal muscles to prepare for flight. Your pupils dilate, allowing for better night vision, and your body consumes more oxygen to fuel these changes. You are ready to enter into mortal combat with the tiger, or more sensibly, run for your life.

After the appropriate burst of physical activity, your body chemistry returns to normal and you can breathe a sigh of relief.

Now open your eyes. Welcome back to the twenty-first century. We are no longer threatened by saber-toothed tigers. It used to be that we had a physical outlet for our stress response—fighting or fleeing for safety. And anyway, Mother Nature wasn't overly concerned with our emotional well-being; staying alive long enough to have children was the main thing. Yet while we no longer spend our days hunting or being hunted and the stressors in our lives are very different, our response to stress remains the same. The death of a close friend or relative, divorce, or the loss of our job can all seem very stressful. A change in financial or personal status, such as retirement (especially if it's forced upon us), or even a positive life change like getting married or moving, can trigger the stress-response system. If this system gets triggered too often, or if we remain under stress for too long, it can cause great harm, especially for those chemically vulnerable to depression. Even if you are not biologically wired for depression, enough stress can bring it on.

It happens in animals. In fact, new antidepressants are first tested by stressing an animal to the point where he becomes depressed. The more effective the antidepressant, the higher the animal's threshold. In one famous test, known as the forced swimming test, a rat supported by a tiny life jacket is placed in a tank full of water. The rat's initial reaction is to try to swim his way out. But since he can't escape, his efforts are for naught. So what happens? The stressed-out animal becomes profoundly depressed and gives up. But if fortified with an antidepressant before being dunked, rats can continue swimming for a much longer period of time before giving up.

Stressed-out humans often react the same way. When life events become unbearable, as hard as we may try to cope we can also become depressed. Like those unfortunate rats, we can tread water for only so long. In fact, some of the worst biological depressions can be triggered by events. Few severely depressed patients come to see me and say, "Gee, everything in my life is great, but I'm miserable." In most cases, the depression has been triggered by some stressful life change. Those with a particular biological vulnerability may have a lower threshold of stress than others, but none of us are immune.

Severely depressed people pour out higher levels of cortisol than normal. Ironically, although they may appear to be slowed down and sluggish, in reality their brains are in overdrive, draining them both physically and emotionally. The continual bombardment of stress hormones in general and cortisol in particular has a devastating effect on all the organs of the body. It eats away at the arteries of the heart, increasing the risk of heart attack and stroke. It can make blood sugar soar to dangerous levels, leading to diabetes. It also makes us more prone to ulcers and osteoporosis. It can even dampen the immune system, making us vulnerable to infections and possibly even cancer.

The brain is particularly vulnerable to the lethal effect of stress hormones out of control. In fact, high levels of cortisol can actually destroy brain cells in the memory center of the brain, the hippocampus. Cortisol may also interfere with the production or uptake of neurotransmitters, which will have an adverse impact on mood. The more episodes of serious depression a person experiences, the less stress it takes to trigger the next episode. Indeed, after a while, it seems that even the most minimal stress can send him or her back into a depressed state. This phenomenon has led researchers to theorize that the brains of depressed people have become sensitized to operating in a depressed way. Some people may have a stress-response system that is overly sensitive. Ironically, these people may have done beautifully in the days when we were stalked by saber-toothed tigers, or they may be sensitive to subtle social nuances, but today their highly sensitized reaction to stress can be a liability.

When Should Depression Be Treated?

If it's becoming increasingly difficult to distinguish between biological depression and so-called event depression, then the question arises, when should depression be treated, and when should it be allowed to "run its course"? If someone is severely depressed, there is no question that they should seek treatment. They are putting their life at risk if they don't.

Mild-to-moderate depression can be transient. If the depression lifts on its own within a few weeks, then treatment may not be necessary. If, however, the depression recurs and is interfering with the quality of life, the right treatment may prevent the depression from worsening down the road.

The question of when to treat depression is particularly difficult to answer in terms of grief. Medical students are still taught that it is wrong to give a grieving person an antidepressant, because it will interfere with the normal grieving process. Many of us who practice psychiatry and see the extent to which people suffer from loss would disagree with this dogma. How and when to treat a patient is a highly individual matter, depending on that person's particular threshold. Some people can recover from a loss fairly quickly. Although they may still be grieving the loss of a loved one, they can return to work and normal living within a few weeks. Others may be paralyzed by the loss. No matter what they do, or how hard they try, they can't lift themselves out of their despair. In these cases, grief has crossed over into biological depression. Once your stress-response system is in overdrive, it is nearly impossible to experience the normal stages of grief. Although it is controversial, I think that in these cases, treatment is the most compassionate and practical approach. Taking SAM-e can help lift you out of the severe depression so that you can begin to deal with the loss in a meaningful way. I want to make one point very clear: Treating your depression is not going to make you happy, but it will give you the strength to better cope with your loss.

A Word to Parents: Nurture Can Win Over Nature

To an extent, biology is destiny, in that those of us born with a genetic tendency to become depressed are at greater risk of experiencing depression at some point. The likelihood of depression is always exacerbated by stressful life events. Yet in many cases, biological vulnerabilities can be overcome. In this regard, we humans can learn an important lesson from the animal kingdom. Monkeys, who have a biochemistry similar to ours, suffer from depression at the same rate as humans and respond equally well to antidepressants. You may ask, how can we tell when monkeys are depressed? The answer is simple: They act like depressed people. A happy monkey is outgoing and appropriately assertive of his rights. A depressed monkey is timid in new situations and allows himself to be pushed around by the others. Like humans, not all monkeys who are born with a genetic predisposition to depression actually become depressed. What might make the difference? One theory is that the style of mothering accounts for it! A monkey reared by an attentive mother who teaches her critical social and coping skills is more likely to turn out just fine. She can rise in the hierarchy of monkey life and pursue what appears to be a fulfilling life (at least for a monkey!). A genetically vulnerable monkey who is not lucky enough to have a good mother will succumb to depression. I think the lesson to be learned here by us humans is that although depression may run in some families, it need not plague every generation. We can't overestimate the importance of a good role model for children in teaching them the coping skills necessary for life. For that reason alone, it is vitally important for parents who are depressed to get the help they need. Depression interferes in countless ways with your ability to be a good, involved parent and role model. Dealing with your depression constructively not only will send a strongly positive message to your children but will improve your ability to parent. It may be the best thing you can do to prevent them from ever having to suffer.

3

The SAM-e Story

"I have a neurological illness that caused depression and memory problems. I've been taking SAM-e for three years. I was lucky. I had relatives in Italy who bought it from a local pharmacy and sent it to me. I feel much better. My mind is sharper. Now I have a lot more energy."

S.G.

"Two weeks after starting SAM-e, I really began to feel better. One excellent gauge of how I feel is that I've been getting a tremendous amount of work done. The increase in my productivity at work has been phenomenal. I went from basically being paralyzed at work, to getting as much done as I need to . . . and more."

M.P.

When people start taking SAM-e for the first time, two things usually happen. Within *days*, their mood begins to lift and they have an increased sense of well-being. But that's not all. They also report something quite unique to SAM-e. They consistently say that they actually feel more energetic and healthier. That's quite a change from what you generally hear from a patient starting an antidepressant.

Unlike other antidepressants, SAM-e is made from substances normally found in the human body—methionine and adenosine triphosphate (or ATP). Methionine is an essential amino acid, a building block of protein. Found in high-protein foods such as meat and fish, methionine is also made in small amounts by our cells, but not in enough quantity to meet the body's needs.

Good nutrition is key to maintaining adequate methionine levels. Here's why. Two key B vitamins, B_{12} and folic acid, are required for the production of methionine. In fact, a deficiency in either one of these vitamins can result in depression and problems in mental function, especially among older people. Much of Terry's research has centered on the role of these B vitamins in depression in general and in the production of SAM-e in particular. As we will explain later, the two are inextricably linked, and the SAM-e story cannot be told without including these vitamins.

ATP is a high-powered fuel that is produced by the cells to provide energy to run the body. It is present in almost every cell and provides the juice to run all of the body's machinery. There is plenty of it to go around.

The product of this marriage of methionine and ATP is SAM-e, a molecule essential to many aspects of human health. But SAM-e levels are not evenly distributed among all humans. Blood levels of SAM-e are seven times higher in children than in adults. Men have slightly higher levels of SAM-e than women do, probably because a considerable amount of SAM-e is produced and consumed in muscle tissue, which is more abundant in men. Levels of SAM-e are notably lower among depressed people of any age.

SAM-e deficiencies are also common in people with neurological problems such as Alzheimer's disease, Parkinson's disease, and HIV complications that can lead to dementia. Terry, who, as noted in Chapter 1, did his Ph.D. on SAM-e in 1982, was one of the first scientists to study this remarkable molecule in connection with the central nervous system and, more specifically, its role in regulating mood and mental function. Recently, Terry discovered that levels of SAM-e are lower in the cerebrospinal fluid of people with neurological complications like depression due to severe vitamin B_{12} or folate deficiency. Low levels of SAM-e in cerebrospinal fluid, as we have seen, indicates an inadequate amount in the brain. Clearly, these are compelling reasons not to let your SAM-e levels fall below normal.

SAM-e Turns On Key Reactions

SAM-e's key role in a process called the methylation cycle makes it absolutely essential for human health. Methylation, a term for a basic yet critical chemical reaction in the body, is the passing of what is known in chemistry as a methyl group—one carbon and three hydrogen atoms—from one molecule to another. Methylation is as vital to human life as breathing. It is an "on-off" switch that activates more than a hundred different processes in the body, from producing important neurotransmitters that allow brain cells to communicate, to preserving bone health, to protecting against heart disease. Methylation activity declines as we age, resulting in a slowdown of these vital activities, which many scientists suspect may contribute to the aging process as well as to the onset of many diseases. There is also compelling evidence that a slowdown in methylation or a genetic tendency to undermethylate may be a key factor in depression for many. There are different kinds of SAM-e/methylation reactions that trigger biological responses throughout the body. These reactions are the "greatest hits" of metabolism. They are what make us alive. When you review the list below, you will see why SAM-e is so fundamental to life that we could not exist without it.

DNA METHYLATION. There is nothing more fundamental to human life than DNA. It's the genetic "software" which runs the cells and contains the genetic code for every living thing. When SAM-e reacts with DNA by donating a methyl group, it allows our genes to spring into action. It's like hitting the "on" switch on a computer; DNA methylation is the operating system of the body, helping it to regulate important processes such as cellular growth and repair, production of immune cells to fight disease, wound healing, and reproduction. The undermethylation of DNA is believed to be a causal factor in cancer, because it could hamper the body's ability to repair damaged cells before they turn cancerous.

PROTEIN METHYLATION. Proteins form the basic structures of many key components of the human body, including muscles, tissues, organs, and even hormones. The methylation of protein is critical for cell growth and repair. Sluggish protein methylation can trigger a downward spiral that can have a devastating impact on the body and mind, leading to deterioration of key organ systems, including the heart and brain. Protein methylation undoubtedly plays a major role in the onset of depression. It is involved in the activation of receptors, special sites on cell membranes which bind with other molecules to stimulate a response—in other words, the body's basic communication system. As discussed in the last chapter, this is especially true of the brain, where sluggish protein metabolism can pitch someone into depression. Studies show that SAM-e supplementation can stimulate protein methylation,

which not only boosts levels of the key neurotransmitters but increases the number of receptors.

PHOSPHOLIPID METHYLATION. Cell membranes are composed of fatlike substances called
phospholipids. In order to get into the cell, substances must first pass through the cell membrane.
As we age, cell membranes can become rigid, making it difficult for vital substances to move in and
out. SAM-e is important for phospholipid methylation, which helps maintain the flexibility of the cell
membrane, keeping it more youthful. Through
methylation, SAM-e also boosts the production of
phosphatidylserine, a phospholipid important for
both mood and memory.

Its role in the methylation cycle places SAM-e at the
heart of many lifesaving functions. But the SAM-e
story doesn't stop here. SAM-e is also essential for another critical process, called trans-sulfuration, which
produces a key chemical, glutathione.

SAM-e Boosts Glutathione

Many of you have heard of antioxidants, a group of
compounds produced by the body and also found in
many different foods, primarily fruits, vegetables,
legumes, and whole grains. Some well-known vitamins
like C, E, and beta carotene are, in fact, antioxidants.
As noted in Chapter 1, antioxidants protect us from

damage caused by highly reactive compounds called free radicals. The human body requires oxygen for its basic chemical functioning, for metabolism, for energy. Everything we do requires energy, both conscious activities like walking and automatic body functions like our heartbeat and breathing. Oxygen is the fuel that drives energy production and makes life possible, but it leaves behind a potentially dangerous by-product—the unstable oxygen molecules called free radicals. Free radicals are fine up to a point—in fact, without them, we couldn't live. If allowed to accumulate, however, they can cause a great deal of mischief. They can attack DNA, possibly initiating cancer. They can attack fat molecules in the blood, causing them to oxidize and form plaque, thereby clogging the arteries. They can target cells in key areas of the brain and may be a factor in brain aging.

The body has a defense system that controls free radicals, and glutathione—known as the "master antioxidant"—is at its heart. You cannot obtain glutathione through diet; it must be produced by the cells. So crucial is it to the body that living a long, healthy life requires making a constant supply. Below is a review of just a few of the lifesaving functions that glutathione performs in the body. It could not perform any of these tasks without SAM-e.

DETOXIFIES THE LIVER. There is a huge amount of glutathione in the liver, which also contains the body's heaviest concentration of SAM-e. The liver has many crucial jobs, including the production of bile, but its most important role is the detoxification of drugs (including the tricyclic antidepressants), alcohol, and poisons that are ingested in food, such as insecticides, or produced by the body through normal metabolism. When glutathione encounters toxic compounds in the liver, it attaches itself to them, making them more water-soluble. This allows the toxins to be flushed out through the kidneys. Liver damage occurs when the liver is so overwhelmed by toxins that it cannot produce enough cleansing glutathione. As I will discuss in Chapter 11 ("Getting Healthy with SAM-e"), SAM-e has been used as an effective treatment for liver disease, especially alcohol-induced liver damage.

PROTECTS DNA. Glutathione protects DNA from damage by free radicals, which can contribute to diseases such as cancer and premature aging.

BOOSTS THE IMMUNE SYSTEM. Glutathione is also important for a well-functioning immune system, the body's defense against disease. Interestingly, several studies have documented a link between depression and weakened immune function. Although it has never been studied, the decline in immunity seen in depression could be related to a scarcity of glutathione caused by a deficiency in SAM-e.

REDUCES INFLAMMATION. Another vital function of glutathione is the role it plays in the reduction of inflammation, which is the primary cause of discomfort in osteoarthritis, a condition caused by the wearing down of the cartilage (the protective covering on bones). As noted, SAM-e is also a highly effective treatment for osteoarthritis, which could be due in part to its glutathione-boosting effect. (For more information on SAM-e and arthritis, see Chapter 11, "Getting Healthy with SAM-e.")

Without SAM-e, the body could not make adequate amounts of glutathione. In the process called transsulfuration, SAM-e helps produce the precursor to glutathione, the amino acid cysteine. Cysteine combines with two other amino acids, glutamic acid and glycine, to form the precious glutathione. Although glutathione is sold as a supplement, there is controversy about whether it can be used by the body in that form. Many scientists believe it breaks down in the stomach before it can reach the bloodstream. Therefore, one of the few *effective* ways to boost glutathione is to take supplemental SAM-e.

In addition to its ability to boost glutathione, SAM-e is also essential for the production of another type of compound found in the body called polyamines. The polyamines spermidine and spermine are involved in cell growth and cell differentiation. They also have an anti-inflammatory effect.

Although SAM-e performs hundreds of roles in the body, its ability to boost glutathione is one of its most important. But there is still more to report on the incredible SAM-e story.

The SAM-e/Homocysteine Connection

Recently, an amino acid called homocysteine has gained notoriety as a recognized risk factor for heart disease, stroke, and even some forms of cancer. What isn't widely known is SAM-e's key role in helping to control homocysteine.

Homocysteine is produced by every cell in the body as a normal part of the methylation cycle. Like free radicals, homocysteine can actually be useful in small amounts, but if allowed to accumulate, it can be terribly dangerous. Folic acid and Vitamin B_{12} can reduce homocysteine by converting it to methionine, the building block of SAM-e. SAM-e, in turn, helps remove homocysteine by increasing the activity of an enzyme (cystathione-beta-synthetase) that converts this potentially harmful amino acid into the beneficial glutathione.

Here's another reason to keep your SAM-e levels high. Low SAM-e levels often go hand in hand with high homocysteine. Even slightly elevated levels of homocysteine are believed to increase the risk of heart disease and other problems:

- Homocysteine is toxic to the endothelial cells that line blood vessels. Damaged endothelial cells may lead to the formation of plaque in the arteries, causing heart attack and stroke.

- Homocysteine may increase the risk of blood clots.
- The Stroke Prevention in Young Women Study revealed that young women with levels of homocysteine in the top tenth percentile had nearly *triple* the risk of stroke—a risk comparable to that of smoking a pack of cigarettes daily.

High levels of homocysteine and a low intake of B vitamins are now believed to be risk factors in several other diseases, including reproductive cancers in women and cancers of the colon. More recently, they have been shown to be risk factors for Alzheimer's dementia.

There is also a link between high levels of homocysteine, low levels of SAM-e, and depression. Terry's research found low levels of folate and SAM-e in the red blood cells and spinal fluid of depressed patients. This was associated with high levels of serum homocysteine. Terry suspects that elevated levels of homocysteine as well as the deficiencies in these key B vitamins may hamper methylation, which could explain their destructive effects on the body and mind.

The homocysteine connection in both heart disease and depression raises some intriguing questions. As noted in Chapter 2, people with depression are at greater risk of developing heart disease, just as people who have heart disease are at risk for depression. In fact, about twenty percent of all heart patients receive a diagnosis of major depression, and as many as one third will have a major depression within one year after their heart attacks. Until recently, the depression associated with heart disease has been dismissed as that which often accompanies any chronic illness. After all, being sick is very stressful and stress is a key trigger for depression; chronic illness is hardly a happy event. However, recent studies show that about half of all patients with heart attacks have had bouts of depression *prior* to the onset of heart disease. Could treating your depression early in life by taking SAM-e prevent heart disease from striking down the road? Although this question has never been studied, we believe it is possible that early intervention could make a difference.

This complicated set of chemical reactions means that SAM-e works on many different systems of the body. As a result, it has been used as a treatment for many different and seemingly unrelated medical problems, including osteoarthritis, liver disease, and fibromyalgia.

SAM-e may help protect the brain against age-related destruction of the cells responsible for mood, memory, and learning. As Terry noted in a recent study published in *Nutrition Reviews* (Vol. 54, No. 12), SAM-e has been shown to be reduced in the cerebrospinal fluid of patients with Alzheimer's dementia, which suggests that methylation in the brain may be important for some forms of dementia. Currently, I am investigating the use of SAM-e as a treatment for Parkinson's disease. (For more information, see Chapter 11, "Getting Healthy with SAM-e".)

The fact that SAM-e is involved in so many different life processes has made it the subject of intense scientific scrutiny. In fact, as noted in Chapter 1, SAM-e has been the subject of thousands of scientific studies, making it the only natural substance to have been so thoroughly researched in both Europe and the United States. In addition to numerous laboratory studies exploring the biochemistry of SAM-e, there have been thirty-nine published clinical studies on the use of SAM-e to control depression. While thirty-nine clinical studies may not seem like a lot, it's actually more than most prescription drugs can boast when they go on the market!

- Close to 1,400 patients have participated in carefully controlled clinical trials on depression alone.
- In several studies directly comparing SAM-e to standard tricyclic medications, SAM-e did as well as or better than these drugs, without the side effects.
- Most of these studies involved severely depressed patients who often did not respond to other antidepressants, but nevertheless did surprisingly well on SAM-e.
- SAM-e has an excellent safety record. It has undergone rigorous testing and is approved as a prescription drug in Italy, Germany, Spain, and Russia.

But what about in the real world? Well, there are hundreds of thousands of patients around the world taking SAM-e for depression. As you know, it outsells

Prozac in Italy. SAM-e's worldwide reputation is excellent, and I have had amazing results with hundreds of patients taking it in my practice.

SAM-e's remarkable antidepressant properties were discovered somewhat serendipitously. Although SAM-e was first identified in 1953, it was not until 1973 that researchers tested it as a treatment for schizophrenia, a disease many believe stems from a glitch in the methylation cycle. While SAM-e did not help to control the symptoms of schizophrenia, researchers were intrigued by one interesting finding. Unexpectedly, the schizophrenic patients treated with SAM-e became less depressed. Since then, scores of studies have investigated SAM-e's role as an antidepressant, and the results have been quite extraordinary.

We're not entirely sure yet how it works, but we do know this: Long-term treatment with SAM-e in animals has been shown to increase brain concentrations of norepinephrine, dopamine, and serotonin. Studies in humans have shown similar results. In one study reported in the journal *The Lancet,* Terry showed that depressed patients treated with SAM-e over a fourteen-day period had a significant increase in cerebrospinal fluid concentrations of a key metabolite that is used as a marker for serotonin levels in the brain. Other researchers have also found that when depressed people are treated with SAM-e, their cerebrospinal fluid levels of the marker for dopamine increase too. The exact way in which SAM-e does this remains unclear, but an increase in these two markers is often associated with antidepressant effect.

Study after study has confirmed that SAM-e excels when tested against a placebo, an important way to test the efficacy of any antidepressant. You may wonder why it is considered important that a drug outperform a placebo, or sugar pill. It may surprise you to learn that at least thirty percent of the effect of any antidepressant—for the first few weeks—is attributed to the so-called placebo effect. In other words, if you believe that a drug will work, it will. Even though the placebo effect wears off within a few weeks, it does underscore the power the mind can hold over the body. Therefore, in order to be certain that a drug and not the placebo effect has brought about a good response, the drug must consistently outperform a placebo by a substantial margin. When matched against a placebo, SAM-e wins hands down.

SAM-e not only outperforms a placebo but can hold its own among other antidepressants. Numerous studies have confirmed that when tested against several of the tricyclic antidepressants, SAM-e does as well, or nearly as well, with virtually no side effects. Also, since with SAM-e few patients drop out because of side effects or delay in onset of action, more people have a chance to respond to it.

Here are some of the research highlights that have advanced our understanding of SAM-e. We've only chosen a few of the many that have been done. (For a more complete list of studies, see the bibliography on page 245.)

THE FIRST SUCCESS. The first double-blind, placebo-controlled study of SAM-e was conducted in 1973 in Verona, Italy. (Neither the researcher nor the patients knew who was taking SAM-e and who was taking the placebo.) Such double-blind, placebo-controlled studies are the gold standard of medical research. The study involved thirty depressed patients ill enough to be in psychiatric hospitals. Twenty of them were given SAM-e for up to fifteen days; the remainder were given a placebo. Based on the Hamilton Rating Scale, the most respected professional index of depression, researchers reported that one hundred percent of the patients— every single one of them—showed improvement in depressed mood while taking SAM-e. Only thirty percent of patients taking the placebo improved. In the researchers' own words, "SAM-e acts favorably and significantly on specific depressive symptoms (depressed mood, work, and interests; suicidal tendencies) which, in a high percentage of patients, were greatly improved." In particular, researchers marveled over how fast SAM-e worked. "The rapid action of the drug should be stressed since in some cases almost all of the symptoms had disappeared after 4 days of treatment, and in general, after 6 or 7 days . . . No untoward side effects were observed

in the patients to whom SAM-e was administered."
(*Journal of Psychiatry Research,* 1976, Vol. 13.)

SAM-E WINS OVER ANOTHER ANTIDEPRESSANT.

Researchers from the University of California's Irvine Medical Center studied eighteen patients suffering from major depression. Nine of the patients were given a two-week course of imipramine, a widely used tricyclic antidepressant. The other nine were given SAM-e for the same length of time. By the end of the fourteenth day, fully two-thirds of the SAM-e patients had shown a significant improvement in depressive symptoms. Only twenty-two percent of the imipramine patients had the same relief. "It appears," concluded the researchers, "that S-adenosylmethionine is a rapid and effective treatment for major depression and has few side effects." Noting that SAM-e worked faster than imipramine, the researchers added, "This characteristic of the drug may be a considerable advantage, considering the known risk of suicide during the early phase of treatment with tricyclic antidepressants." In other words, because it works so quickly, in some cases SAM-e could make the difference between life and death. (*American Journal of Psychiatry,* "S-Adenosylmethionine Treatment of Depression: A Controlled Clinical Trial," September 1988, 145:9.)

SAM-E AT MASS GENERAL.

Researchers at Harvard University's affiliated Massachusetts General

Hospital studied the effect of SAM-e on twenty patients, nine of whom had been classified as treatment-resistant because they did not improve on other antidepressants. The patients were given oral doses of SAM-e for up to six weeks. Researchers noted, "The group as a whole significantly improved with oral SAM-e." Of the eleven patients who were not treatment-resistant, seven showed a full antidepressant response on the Hamilton Rating Scale (an improvement of fifty percent or better). Two others showed major improvement but did not achieve a full response. Even more surprising, two of the nine treatment-resistant patients showed a *full* antidepressant response. Considering that very little works with treatment-resistant patients—people for whom standard antidepressants have been ineffective—this is an excellent result. What makes SAM-e's performance even more significant is the fact that not one patient dropped out of the study because of side effects. (*Acta Psychiatry Scandanavica,* "The Antidepressant Potential of Oral S-Adenosyl-l-Methionine," 1990:81, 432–36.)

A MAJOR STUDY'S EXCELLENT RESULTS. A major multicenter study evaluated SAM-e in 195 outpatients in Italy. The subjects were given daily 400mg injections of SAM-e for fifteen days. At the end of the study, 163 patients were evaluated (the rest were excluded either for lack of compliance or because it was determined that they did not meet the criteria to participate in the study in the first place). The senior researcher, Dr. Maurizio Fava of the Depression Research Center of Harvard's Massachusetts General Hospital, and his Italian coresearchers reported that depressive symptoms were significantly reduced after seven days for more than half of the patients who completed the study. In fact, ninety patients showed more than a fifty percent improvement on standard assessment tests. This is considered an excellent result. No severe side effects were reported, an encouraging and unusual finding for such a large study involving an antidepressant. (*Journal of Psychiatry Research*, 1995:56, 295–97.)

DESIPRAMINE OUTPERFORMED BY SAM-E!

In 1994, a research team headed by Kate M. Bell at the University of California, Irvine Medical Center compared SAM-e with desipramine, a tricyclic antidepressant. Twenty-six patients were involved in a double-blind study comparing oral SAM-e with oral desipramine. At the end of four weeks, sixty-two percent of the patients taking SAM-e and fifty percent of the patients taking desipramine showed significant improvement.

The researchers also investigated whether there was a correlation between blood levels of SAM-e and mood. One interesting finding: Regardless of which drug they took, patients showing a fifty percent improvement or better in the Hamilton Rating Scale score—which is considered a full response, an excellent result—had a significant increase in blood plasma levels of SAM-e. As the researchers noted, "We found a significant relationship between change in plasma SAM-e concentration and clinical improvement. . . . In summary, the significant correlation between plasma SAM-e levels and the degrees of clinical improvement regardless of the type of treatment suggests that SAM-e might play an important role in regulating mood."

THE CHRONICALLY ILL HELPED BY SAM-E.

As noted earlier, depression and illness often go hand in hand. But many people who are ill cannot tolerate antidepressants, or may experience particularly bad side effects from drug interactions. As the researchers in this study noted, in some cases, as with some forms of heart disease, antidepressants may make the chronic illness worse. "The 20 cardiovascular patients in our study were regarded as high-risk subjects because developing depression may cause suicidal ideation with further deterioration of quality of life. Tricyclics and monoamine oxidase . . . inhibitors may be detrimental to cardiac patients because of their toxic cardiovascular side effects." It's a catch-22: Treating severe depression may not only hurt the quality of life but also be life-threatening, yet treating with standard antidepressants may bring about the same result. For these people, SAM-e may be the treatment of choice. Forty-eight patients with major depression and concurrent serious illnesses were given up to 800mg of SAM-e daily. The results as described by the researchers were excellent: "Response of patients treated with SAM-e was quite rapid and many were still improving at the end of the 28-day trial." As noted, patients not only improved quickly on SAM-e, but did not experience any untoward side effects that could worsen their preexisting medical problems. (*Current Therapeutic Research,* June 1994, Vol. 55, No. 6.)

A MAJOR REVIEW OF THE STUDIES. A meta-analysis, a major review of the published clinical studies on SAM-e, published in *Acta Scandinavica Neurologica* in 1994 assessed the efficacy of SAM-e in the treatment of depression. What makes this study so important is that *all* of the clinical trials of SAM-e published between 1973 and 1992 were analyzed. In eleven studies, SAM-e was tested against a placebo. In fourteen studies, SAM-e was tested against a standard prescription antidepressant. In another thirteen studies known as open studies, SAM-e was given to depressed patients without testing it against either a placebo or an antidepressant. The patients were monitored to assess improvement. In every study involving placebos, SAM-e was found to be more effective than the placebo. In fact, the author of the study notes that SAM-e does better on the placebo test than most other prescription antidepressants! In every study involving prescription drugs, SAM-e was found to be as effective as tricyclic antidepressants. In the open studies, patients also showed significant improvement. The review study concluded, "In summary, this meta-analysis shows that the efficacy of SAM-e in treating depressive syndromes and disorders is superior to that of placebo and is comparable to that of standard tricyclic antidepressants. Since SAM-e is a naturally occurring compound with relatively few side-effects, its antidepressant effect makes it a potentially important tool in the armamentarium of the modern psychopharmacologist."

TWO MULTICENTER STUDIES. In a 1997 review article published in *Expert Opinion in Investigational Drugs,* Terry outlined SAM-e's potential as a treatment for psychiatric and neurological disorders. He reported on two as yet unpublished clinical trials on SAM-e conducted at several research centers in Europe involving 197 severely depressed patients (based on the Hamilton Rating Scale). In the first study, involving seventy-five patients, SAM-e was tested against a placebo. Both compounds were given intravenously. Patients taking SAM-e had an average improvement rate of 40.8 percent compared to patients taking the placebo, who improved by only 27.6 percent. Considering how severely ill these patients were, this is an excellent result.

In the second study, SAM-e went head-to-head with clomipramine, perhaps the strongest drug in the antidepressant arsenal. Although clomipramine is highly effective, recovery often comes at the cost of terrible side effects. In fact, many patients simply won't stay on the drug. In the trial, 122 patients were given either SAM-e or clomipramine intravenously for three weeks. Patients taking SAM-e had an average improvement rate of 36.5 percent compared to 48.8 percent for the patients on clomipramine. Even though SAM-e did not outperform clomipramine, it did bring about a major improvement in these severely depressed patients, and it achieved this good result with virtually no side effects. As Terry noted in his review, "The drug-related adverse events and dropouts for adverse events were significantly lower in SAM-e than in clomipramine." In other words, many patients did not continue to take clomipramine, because they could not tolerate the side effects. If the dropouts had been factored into the final result as nonresponders, clomipramine would not have fared as well.

From these studies, it's apparent that although SAM-e may be a powerful antidepressant, it works gently in the body. SAM-e can hold its own among even the strongest of the prescription drugs, yet it does not have any of the onerous side effects.

In the next chapter, we will review the latest information on prescription antidepressants.

4

The Antidepressant Arsenal: What Works, What Doesn't, What's Best for You

Over the past twenty years, the patient-doctor relationship has undergone a major change; a change which, in both Terry's and my opinions, is for the better. Patients are no longer content to be relegated to a passive role with little or no say in their treatment. They expect to be involved and active participants in their recovery, which is how we believe medicine ought to be practiced. I never hand out a prescription without first making sure that my patients know what they taking, why they are taking it, and the potential side effects. In a way, SAM-e is the perfect realization of this philosophy of ours. It puts the power to heal right in the patient's hand.

In Chapter 3, we went into great detail about Terry's work and the rest of the research on SAM-e. From that base, you can see why we feel it is such a unique and effective antidepressant for "gray zone" to moderate depression. It promotes healing quickly, effectively, and without side effects.

But SAM-e is not the whole antidepressant story. SAM-e is just one—albeit a very good one—among a whole arsenal of depression fighters. Each has its own strengths and weaknesses, but I think you'll agree after reading this chapter that SAM-e is the first thing you should turn to when depression strikes.

Antidepressants are a relatively recent phenomenon in modern medicine; they were not in wide use until the 1960s. This is not to say that no one treated depression before then. Traditional Chinese healers often used herbs such as ginkgo biloba to treat depression. Ginkgo helps to promote circulation to the brain and may boost levels of neurotransmitters. The newly rediscovered herb St. John's wort has been used for hundreds of years in Europe for the treatment of what we would now diagnose as depression. Numerous other methods—from herbs to just plain talking—have been used since time began to help treat a condition as much a part of being human as breathing.

People have also found a couple of simple ways to self-medicate their mood disorders. Alcoholic beverages were undoubtedly used for thousands of years—as they still are today—as a way to relieve anxiety and depression, often exacerbating the problem in the process. Smoking has also been used as a means to relieve depression. Studies have shown that people who have the most difficulty quitting smoking are those with a personal or family history of depression. In fact, one of the newest treatments for smoking is an antidepressant marketed under the name Zyban.

During the first half of the twentieth century, Western medicine focused on the new world of psychotherapy, which explored the psychological factors involved in depression, but also used biological methods to treat depression. For most people, psychotherapy will do some good, but it is often inadequate on its own. The other main treatment was electroconvulsive therapy (ECT), also known as shock treatment, in which electrodes are attached to the head and a series of electrical shocks are delivered to the brain. Still performed today, ECT is highly effective, with an eighty to ninety percent success rate in cases of severe depression. Although it is not painful—the patient is anesthetized during the procedure—many patients are concerned about undergoing what sounds scarier than it really is. Popular movies and misconceptions have made the procedure even less appealing. It is also time-consuming, and can take from six to twelve treatments. The main side effect of ECT is a temporary loss of memory, which can be distressing. Obviously, if given a choice between taking a pill or getting shock therapy, most people prefer taking a pill. ECT is now a treatment of last resort, used only for severely depressed patients who have not responded to medication.

The battle against depression underwent a change in the 1950s with the introduction of the first effective antidepressant drug. Iproniazid, a monoamine oxidase inhibitor, was the first of these antidepressants. Initially it was developed as a new treatment for tuberculosis. Although ineffective for tuberculosis, this MAO inhibitor had an unexpected side effect: it boosted the mood of tuberculosis patients, many of whom suffer from depression. In the 1960s, the first tricyclic antidepressant hit the market, and the antidepressant revolution began. Since then, dozens of new antidepressants have appeared.

There is no perfect antidepressant; nothing works consistently well for everybody, all the time. The best of them don't work for nearly a third of the people who try them. Even the much lauded SRIs like Prozac and its cousins aren't perfect. As you'll see, they have significant drawbacks. We think that SAM-e is as close to perfect as it gets. Yet there will be people, primarily those who are severely depressed, who still need to take something else. If you are on a medication that does not work for you, or causes untoward side effects, you may need to change your dose, or try a different drug. You may need to try several before you find the one that's right for you. Remember to check with your doctor before altering anything to do with your prescription antidepressant regimen. As you'll see, these can be very tricky drugs. The point is, don't get discouraged and assume that your case is hopeless. The overwhelming majority of depressions can be helped as long as the patient and doctor persevere.

A case in point is my patient Brian, a business executive who had been struggling with depression for nearly two decades. Brian described himself as a "high-functioning depressive"; that is, although he was depressed, he was able to keep up with his work and family responsibilities. "It was never a matter of whether or not an antidepressant would work for me—I could never stay on one long enough to find out," Brian recalled. "When I tried Prozac six years ago, I developed every side effect in the book from insomnia to sexual dysfunction and anxiety attacks. I had the same bad side effects from nortriptyline and nefazodone. I tried yet another antidepressant that produced hallucinations. After that I said no more drugs. I was reconciled to living with my depression."

But recently, a sudden business reversal sent Brian into a paralyzing depression, the worst he had ever experienced. "I was going down, down, down, with no end in sight," Brian said. "I couldn't work, I couldn't function."

Faced with the prospect of remaining paralyzed, Brian agreed to try one more antidepressant. This time it was SAM-e. "After taking SAM-e for a few days, I began to feel better. I'm not saying that I was instantly happy or euphoric, but I was no longer in despair. There were absolutely no side effects, which was a real surprise. Within a short time, I was able to get back to work, which to me was very important. Now I'm still taking SAM-e and I feel reasonably good."

Brian's experience is all too typical; patients often find that they cannot tolerate the side effects of standard antidepressants. In the following pages, I will review the other commonly prescribed antidepressants used in modern medicine. Reading this chapter will help you to better understand why SAM-e is such an important addition to the antidepressant arsenal.

Tricyclic Antidepressants

THE BASICS

Because of the potential for problems with MAO inhibitors, tricyclic antidepressants are used much more often. There are several different types of tricyclics and a dizzying array of names. The most common are marketed under the names Elavil (amitriptyline), Tofranil (imipramine), Pamelor (nortriptyline), Sinequan (doxepin), Norpramin (desipramine), and Anafranil (clomipramine). While tricyclics are easier to dose than MAO inhibitors, they can cause some unpleasant side effects. You should also know that nonpsychiatrists tend to prescribe doses of tricyclics that may be too low to be effective. I advise patients to be under the care of a psychiatrist when taking tricyclics. If you are not experiencing a full recovery from your depression, it is important to let your doctor know. He or she may need to increase the dose or select another drug. On the other hand, even a modest overdose of tricyclics can be fatal.

It takes about a month for these drugs to have a noticeable effect on mood. The onset of effectiveness can be accelerated by combining it with SAM-e. Again, check with your doctor before altering your prescription drug pattern. Incidentally, if your doctor is over forty-five, he or she is more likely to prescribe a tricyclic than younger doctors who began practicing medicine after the introduction of Prozac and other selective serotonin reuptake inhibitors (SRIs).

Studies estimate most tricyclics to be effective in about seventy percent of cases. However, these numbers do not take into account the high percentage of people who have dropped out of studies because of intolerable side effects. When that is factored in, the real-world effectiveness of tricyclic antidepressants is much lower.

SIDE EFFECTS

Tricyclics are an improvement over the MAO inhibitors in that they are not as risky to take. (See page 98.) But they are still dangerous drugs which can be fatal. Many of the side effects associated with tricyclics stem from their effect on the neurotransmitter acetylcholine—the same action that makes them effective in the first place. Drugs such as the tricyclics which inhibit the action of acetylcholine work against the cholinergic nerves, which control many glandular functions throughout the body, including the production of saliva and mucus. As a result, dry mouth, dry eyes, dry vagina, and constipation are common complaints for people taking tricyclics. Although these side effects are not life-threatening, they can certainly put a crimp in your lifestyle. Chewing gum, using special lubricating drops for the eyes, and using lubricants for vaginal dryness can help relieve those problems to some extent. Eating more fiber and drinking at least eight glasses of water daily can help maintain bowel function. For many people, weight gain is a major problem, not to mention nausea and perpetual drowsiness. Some people complain of feeling "drugged." Tricyclics can also cause a sharp drop in blood pressure. Some of these side effects can be ameliorated by lowering the dosage, which may be possible if SAM-e is added to the treatment regimen.

CAUTIONS

Elderly people in particular are sensitive to the anticholinergic activity of the tricyclics. Tricyclics can cause urinary hesitation or retention, which makes them a bad choice for older men with benign prostate hypertrophy (BPH), who are already prone to urinary difficulties. They can also cause loss of bladder control in both sexes. Moreover, the blood pressure issue makes fainting and falling a real risk in older people.

PERSONAL OBSERVATIONS

The first month of taking a tricyclic can be rough for patients, particularly since they must cope with their depression plus new side effects. Remember that a hallmark of depression is a dark, pessimistic view of the future, and then imagine what that first month is like. The future must seem even blacker than before—you are depressed *and* suffering major side effects. Once the depression begins to lift, however, patients have fewer complaints. I think the side effects are still there, but as patients feel better, they are more willing to put up with them. If the side effects remain unbearable but the patient must continue on these drugs, it may be possible, as noted above, to cut back on the dose, thereby reducing side effects, by adding SAM-e to the treatment regimen.

Selective Serotonin Reuptake Inhibitors (SRIs)

THE BASICS

In the 1950s, researchers discovered the presence of serotonin, one of the "big three" neurotransmitters in the brain. They noticed that low levels of serotonin corresponded with suicidal behavior, leading them to suspect that it was a key factor in depression. The selective serotonin reuptake inhibitors are a class of drugs that prevent the uptake of serotonin by the neurotransmitters, allowing more serotonin to accumulate in the synaptic spaces (the gaps between neurons). The first SRI, Prozac (fluoxetine), appeared in 1988 to much fanfare. At first blush, it seemed like the last word on depression. By 1989, it was one of the top-selling drugs in the United States and it still is. It now has to share some of its market with newer SRIs, including Paxil (paroxetine), Zoloft (sertraline), Luvox (fluvoxamine), and Celexa (citalopram), which are similar in action. (Zoloft is different in that, like SAM-e, it also boosts levels of dopamine, another important neurotransmitter.) The newest SRI-like drug on the block is Effexor (venlafaxine), which is often prescribed for people for whom the other SRIs don't work. In addition to depression, SRIs are prescribed for other psychiatric problems including eating disorders, schizophrenia, obsessive-compulsive disorders, and social phobias. These drugs take from four to twelve weeks to achieve full effect. Once again, the effect can be accelerated by adding SAM-e to the treatment regimen— but please, check with your doctor before altering anything to do with your prescription drug schedule.

As with tricyclics, SRIs don't work for everybody. The studies evaluating their effectiveness have also had a high dropout rate due to side effect intolerance. So while conventional wisdom says this class of drugs ought to work in over seventy percent of cases, the reality is more discouraging.

SIDE EFFECTS

The side effects of SRIs tend to be less intense than those of either the MAO inhibitors or the tricyclics. Initially, patients may complain of headache, nausea, diarrhea, and, perversely, anxiety. Some complain of fatigue. SRIs can cause sleep disturbances called microawakenings, minor sleep disruptions which can interfere with the quality of sleep. The more serious and troubling problems tend to strike down the road. Weight gain is one of them. At first, patients may lose a few pounds, but within six months to a year, many begin to put on a considerable amount of weight. Given the fact that our culture is so weight-conscious, putting on an extra ten to twenty pounds within a year can be very upsetting—especially for women—and can have significant long-term health risks. In addition, some women experience painful breast enlargement.

Sexual dysfunction is the primary complaint of people taking SRIs. In fact, about seventy percent of patients will complain of a loss of interest in sex, difficulty in arousal, lubrication problems or difficulty having an erection, and inhibition of orgasm. In general, this not only is personally distressing but can cause a great strain in intimate relationships. (Because SRIs inhibit orgasm, they are useful for the treatment of premature ejaculation.) Unless these sexual problems are discussed—which they often are not—it is not unreasonable for partners to think that their loved ones have lost interest in them. Generally, sexual problems are not noticed until several months into the treatment; during the first few weeks after the drug starts to work, people are focused on climbing out of depression and returning to normal function. But understandably, as life begins to return to normal, the sexual problems become an acute concern. While the dimensions of this problem are still emerging, sexual side effects are probably the number one reason why people stop taking SRIs and switch to another medication. For patients with severe depression, I have been able to reduce side effects by cutting the dose and adding SAM-e to the treatment regimen.

CAUTIONS

Although SRIs are not as likely to cause problems with drug interactions as the MAO inhibitors, there are some drugs that you should not take while taking an SRI. Be sure that your doctor has given you a complete list. You must wait at least two weeks after discontinuing an SRI (and five weeks if you are taking Prozac) to take an MAO inhibitor. The most commonly used drug of all, alcohol, can greatly exacerbate the sedative effect of an SRI. I had a patient on Prozac who after drinking a martini at a dinner party literally passed out midsentence over (actually into) the soup course! His wife was there to rescue him, and although it was embarrassing, the consequences would have been far more serious had he been behind the wheel of a car. As a general rule, SRIs and alcohol don't mix. In fact, psychotropic drugs and alcohol don't mix.

PERSONAL OBSERVATIONS

Psychiatry errs on the side of downplaying the sexual side effects of SRIs, to the disservice of our patients.

Although I knew that sexual dysfunction was a common complaint among patients taking these drugs, I, like most doctors, tried to minimize it. After all, sexual dysfunction was less important than relieving your depression. I did not fully understand the magnitude of this problem until 1994, when I was a guest on a national cable TV show addressing the sexual problems of people taking Prozac. During the first half hour of the show, the switchboard lit up with more than fifteen thousand calls from around the country. Countless others tried to get through but couldn't. People felt that their doctors were dismissive of their complaints, as I had been. In some cases, patients said they were reluctant to discuss these personal details with their doctors. As noted, more women take antidepressants than men, but I would wager that most of the studies on the effect of antidepressants are conducted by men. Women may not feel like discussing the intimate details of their sex lives with a man, especially if he is not their primary doctor. It is often not a comfortable environment in which to answer truthfully questions such as, "Have you lost interest in sex?" or, "Are you having difficulty becoming aroused and lubricated?" Another problem is the fact that many of these studies track patients for only the first few weeks in which they are taking an antidepressant. Since sexual side effects are generally not a problem until several months or even a year later, they are simply not picked up. As a result, I believe these problems are dramatically underreported in the clinical trials.

Other Prescription Drugs

THE BASICS

Three other antidepressants which can't be classified into any one group have also proven to be useful: Wellbutrin (bupropion), Serzone (nefazodone), and Remeron (mirtazapine). They are not nearly as well known or widely used as the SRIs or tricyclics—they are not marketed as aggressively—yet they can be good choices for some people. In early studies, Wellbutrin was shown to slightly increase the risk of seizure at higher doses, a problem that can also occur with some tricyclics. Although with proper dosage this should not be a problem, many doctors are still reluctant to prescribe this drug. Marketed under the name Zyban, Wellbutrin can help to break the smoking habit. This is not surprising; as we have seen, studies have shown that smokers who are recidivists (that is, they've tried to quit but can't) typically have a high rate of depression. However, many antidepressants have not worked as smoking cessation aids.

SIDE EFFECTS

There are fewer side effects for these drugs than for the others discussed here. They do not usually cause sexual problems as SRIs do, but patients may complain of nausea, insomnia, and gastrointestinal problems like diarrhea. When compared to SAM-e, they still cause many more side effects.

PERSONAL OBSERVATIONS

These drugs have far fewer anticholinergic effects than the tricyclics, making them a good choice for older people who may not respond well to SRIs. I have found that Wellbutrin in particular is a good drug for older people because it seems not only to enhance well-being but to have an energizing effect similar to SAM-e. Of course, as noted earlier, it must be carefully dosed to avoid the risk of seizure. Since SAM-e is nontoxic even at high doses, I believe it is a better choice.

Monoamine Oxidase Inhibitors

THE BASICS

Monoamine oxidase inhibitors (MAO inhibitors or MAOs) are a class of drugs which include Nardil (phenelzine), Parnate (tranylcypromine), Marplan (iso-carboxazid), and Eldepryl (selegiline). Somewhat rare in the United States, they are prescribed for severe depression, atypical (episodic) depression, and panic disorders. As described in Chapter 2, MAOs inhibit the activity of the monoamine oxidase enzyme, preventing it from breaking down neurotransmitters at the synapse. As a result, they boost levels of noradrenaline and serotonin, key neurotransmitters involved in mood and brain function. MAO inhibitors are powerful but difficult-to-manage drugs; they should only be used under the supervision of an experienced psychopharmacologist. Overdoses can be fatal, and misdoing is easy. MAOs are used only when all other medications have failed.

SIDE EFFECTS

MAO inhibitors have extremely unpleasant side effects: dizziness, weight gain, fluid retention, insomnia, stomach upset, headaches, sexual dysfunction, fatigue, and anxiety, to name only the major ones. In fact, the side effects can be so severe that unless patients are severely debilitated by their depression, they often flat-out refuse to continue taking these drugs.

CAUTIONS

MAO inhibitors can interact adversely with other medications; they should not be used with SAM-e or any other antidepressant. While taking these drugs, and for two weeks following their discontinuation, patients must heed the following advice:

Beware prescription drugs. As a rule, patients should not combine MAO inhibitors with other medication unless specifically instructed by their psychopharmacologist. MAO inhibitors are particularly dangerous in combination with beta-blockers, levodopa, sulfa drugs, sumatriptan, and other commonly prescribed drugs. Get a complete list from your doctor.

No cold medicines! Patients must also avoid over-the-counter cold medicines with ingredients such as phenylpropanolamine, dextromethorphan, pseudoephedrine, and ephedrine, which in combination with MAO inhibitors can cause a steep rise in blood pressure. Also avoid herbal cold remedies containing ephedra or ma huang.

Avoid forbidden foods. People taking MAO inhibitors must avoid foods containing the amine tyramine, which can enhance the effect of the drug and elevate blood pressure to dangerously high levels. There are many foods you should avoid, so be sure to get a complete list from your doctor! Here is a partial list:

- Do not drink any alcoholic beverages no matter how low the alcoholic content.
- Do not eat cheese.
- Do not eat overripe or fermented foods, soy sauce, yeast extracts, bean curd, chicken liver, or processed meats.

If you are taking an MAO inhibitor, you cannot let your guard down, not even once! Recently, I heard the particularly tragic story of a man who had been taking an MAO inhibitor without incident for several years.

One day he got a cold and, without first checking with his doctor, took an over-the-counter cold medicine. Within a few hours, he had died from a stroke. It is critical to keep a list of foods and drugs to avoid posted at home and work. Obviously, MAO inhibitors are not a good choice for most people.

St. John's Wort

THE BASICS

Known by the botanical name *Hypericum perforatum*, Saint John's wort has been popularized as the herbal alternative to prescription antidepressants. Legend has it that this plant sprang from John the Baptist's blood when he was beheaded, hence its odd name. In fact, if you rub the petals of its flower between your fingers, a red resin will ooze out, leaving a stain on your hand. Since ancient times, St. John's wort has been valued as a medicinal herb, not just for depression but for the treatment of ulcers, tumors, and even menstrual cramps. We don't know much about how or why this herb works when compared to the tricyclics and SRIs. Although it is plant-based, it is a far more complicated chemical compound than SAM-e. One major active ingredient in St. John's wort is hyperforin, but there may be other active chemicals as well. Animal studies have shown that, like the SRIs, St. John's wort extract can inhibit the reabsorption of serotonin at the synapse. It also has antiviral and antifungal activity and is being studied as a potential treatment for AIDS and cancer. Recently, St. John's wort has been rediscovered in the United States as a treatment for mild depression. A 1996 study published in the *British Medical Journal* reviewed twenty-three clinical trials involving St. John's wort and concluded that it worked better than a placebo in treating mild-to-moderate depression. This study claimed that it performed almost as well as prescription antidepressants.

The research on St. John's wort, including that reviewed in the *British Medical Journal* study mentioned above, has many problems, among them a shortage of rigorous, published, peer review studies. There is no doubt that in low doses, St. John's wort does have a weak antidepressant effect. It has been tested against tricyclic drugs and has been shown to be as effective. However, the doses of tricyclics in these studies were much lower (50 to 75 mg daily) than what is used in real life. When tested against an effective therapeutic dose of the tricyclic imipramine (150mg daily), as SAM-e has been repeatedly, six pills daily of St. John's wort—double the usual dose—was close in effectiveness. It wasn't as good, but it was close. In fact, at these high doses—the kind required to treat most depression—St. John's wort can have side effects similar to Prozac. And like SRIs, St. John's wort can take from four to twelve weeks to be fully effective. Due to the herb's growing popularity, the National Institutes of Health has recently begun the first U.S. clinical trial of St. John's wort.

From a clinical perspective, SAM-e is stronger and more effective than St. John's wort, with fewer side effects. In some cases, I combine SAM-e with St. John's wort for patients who have not fully responded to either antidepressant.

SIDE EFFECTS

Yes! Despite what you may have heard, St. John's wort can cause side effects similar to those of the SRIs, including jitteriness, loose bowels, jaw clenching, and sexual dysfunction. Since the popularity of St. John's wort has increased, I have had many referrals from physicians whose patients developed sexual side effects while taking it. Because St. John's wort is touted as side-effect-free—and because it is an herb—no one expected it to cause problems. St. John's wort may also cause photosensitivity in fair-skinned people. If you are taking this herb, it is probably wise to limit your time in direct sunlight, especially during the peak burning hours of ten A.M. to two P.M.

When St. John's wort was first introduced to the United States, some researchers assumed that it was similar in action to MAO inhibitors. Therefore, they recommended that people taking St. John's wort avoid the same foods and drugs as they would on an MAO inhibitor. This is simply not true.

CAUTIONS

Do not use St. John's wort with an MAO inhibitor.

PERSONAL OBSERVATIONS

Despite my belief that St. John's wort has been over-rated, there are some people who might benefit from it, notably those who have responded to a low dose of an SRI but could not tolerate the side effects. I have also recommended St. John's wort to patients who absolutely refused to even consider taking a prescription medication, but felt comfortable taking an herbal supplement. I suspect that they, and people like them, will switch to SAM-e once it becomes widely available.

Part 2

Three
Simple Ways
to Stop Depression

5

The Safe and Simple Stop Depression Now Program

If treating depression were as simple as taking a pill—even a pill as good as SAM-e—all psychiatrists would be out of business. And while that would be a wonderful thing for depression sufferers everywhere, it is just not realistic. No, an effective depression treatment must be part of an integrated plan. It must involve medicine, diet, and the power of the mind, body, and spirit.

This is not to say that SAM-e isn't a powerful treatment for depression. It is the best treatment to come along in years. It works faster, better, and without side effects.

But SAM-e can't do it alone.

You must help. That is why the Stop Depression Now program places equal importance on diet and lifestyle.

When I trained to be a psychiatrist, the medical profession still minimized the power of the individual to change. This was the heyday of talk therapy and we were taught that only it—and to a lesser extent, tricyclic antidepressants—could treat clinical depression. We thought that lifestyle and diet had nothing to do with it, and to suggest otherwise was quackery.

Slowly we've awakened to the power of our actions, our habits, and our thoughts.

Just fifty years ago, doctors had no idea that exercise and diet were inextricably linked to heart disease, but now we almost take that for granted. Well, depression is no different. Just as a heart patient needs medicine, a healthy diet, and the right lifestyle, so a depressed person needs the right antidepressant, the right diet, and a depression-proof life. Then you can stop your depression quickly . . . and maybe even permanently. In order to make this process as simple and user-friendly as possible, we've designed a four-step program to get you better.

Obviously, taking SAM-e is the key step in this program. Learning how and when to take the right dose for you and what you can expect from it is the point of Chapter 6 ("How to Take SAM-e"). I suspect it will be the chapter you refer to most often in the beginning. That is how it should be.

Why?

Because depression steals your ability to rebound. It steals your will to change, and saps your strength for healing. That's why the first step you'll take in fighting depression is SAM-e. SAM-e will stop your depression *fast*. Then you can attend to the changes that will lift it completely and keep it away for good. SAM-e is the catalyst for healing. It gives you the vision to see life more clearly. When you begin to feel better, you realize that things just seem different than they seemed when you were depressed. This perspective, this changing attitude, gives you the ability to start making positive changes in your life.

Four Steps
to Stop Depression Now

STEP 1. ASSESS YOUR MOOD

You'd be horrified if you took your car into the shop and the mechanic started repairing things before he even found out what was wrong. You'd probably be just as horrified if you went to the doctor and he gave you a prescription without even hearing your complaint! Well, it's equally foolish to start treating your depression without an assessment of where you are—a self-diagnosis, if you will.

You may remember that earlier we referred to depression as the common cold of psychiatric ailments because it is so widespread. It may be widespread, but it's not always easy to recognize the symptoms of depression. The signs are often subtle and can easily be overlooked, unless you know what to look for.

In order to help you recognize the signs of a depression, we have included in Chapter 6 a useful self-test for assessing your mood, the Depression Severity Scale. This test requires no fancy mathematics or extensive interpretation. Answering the simple questions truthfully will help you to better understand your depression:

- 0–5 Not depressed
- 6–12 Gray zone
- 13–18 Mild-to-moderate depression
- 19–27 Severe depression

Knowing where you fit on this scale will allow you to find the right dose of SAM-e for you.

After you've been taking SAM-e for a little while, you'll come back to this assessment to evaluate your progress and readjust your dose. Throughout your journey out of depression, this self-test will act as a milestone, telling you just how far you've come.

STEP 2. TAKE SAM-E

You've already heard a great deal about SAM-e: how it was discovered, why it works, what the research says, and how it can help you. I don't think you need any more convincing that SAM-e is the key to this depression-fighting program.

So, in this step you'll learn how to take your SAM-e. Drawing on both the voluminous research and my own clinical experience in treating with SAM-e, Chapter 6 will give you some easy guidelines to follow.

DOSAGE. *How much SAM-e do you need?* We'll base your dose on your score from the self-assessment. The vast majority of you will do fine on 400mg a day, but some of you may require as much as 800mg. After a while, as noted, you'll retest yourself and readjust your dose accordingly.

TIME. *How long until SAM-e starts to work, and how long will you need to take it?* There are no hard-and-fast answers for either of these questions. Most people start to feel better just seven days after beginning to take SAM-e; some may respond even faster. How long you must remain on SAM-e is a more difficult issue. It depends on how often you've been depressed over the course of your life, and the likelihood of a recurrence.

DETAILS. *What time of day do you take SAM-e? What kind of SAM-e is best?* Determining when you take your SAM-e will be a trial-and-error process for you. Some of you may like the energy boost SAM-e gives you in the afternoon. I'll tell you what most of my patients have done, but ultimately you'll have to decide what works best for you. As far as the kind of SAM-e is concerned, Terry and I will give you some hints learned from both my practice and his research that can help you make sure you are getting the best product available.

STEP 3. EAT THE RIGHT FOOD

As mentioned previously, in addition to studying SAM-e, Terry has devoted years of research to the role of diet and B vitamins in the regulation of mood. In fact, he has made a significant contribution to the understanding of eating habits and depression. His research is conclusive: Eating the right food is crucial to beating depression. We might not want to dwell on it, but chemistry is crucial to our well-being. Like it or not, we are what we eat.

In Chapter 7 ("The Stop Depression Now Food Plan"), you'll learn how to make sure that what you are putting into your body keeps you as healthy as possible. Paying attention to which foods can make you feel better and which ones will make you blue can save a lot of anguish later. The Stop Depression Now food plan feeds your mental—and physical—health.

Food isn't always enough, though. As you've seen, Terry's research showed low SAM-e levels in the cerebrospinal fluid of depressed people. This goes a long way toward proving that SAM-e deficiency is a significant part of the problem. Similarly, other vitamin deficiencies (or simply less-than-optimal levels) can have a profound impact on your mood. There are also specific supplements you can take to make your SAM-e work even better. Armed with this information, you'll be able to design a supplement regimen that will help you stop depression—and keep it at bay.

STEP 4. ADOPT THE RIGHT LIFESTYLE

Remember, in the beginning of this chapter, I told you that you had to help SAM-e work? Here is where your help comes into play. Antidepressants—and this is true of all of them, not just SAM-e—serve as catalysts to healing. They jump-start the process of getting well. They get you over the hump of depression and give you the energy and drive to keep yourself depression-free.

In order to do that, you will have to learn a new way of thinking and perceiving. Once you begin to repair the chemical imbalance that led to your depression, your new outlook falls naturally into place. This does not mean you need not work at it. You'll find it all too easy to slip into the old mind-set, and you must strive to put what you've learned into practice in your life.

That's the reason for Chapter 8 ("A Simple Guide to Depression-Proofing Your Life"). No one's life stands still for very long, and our mental health depends on how well we take those corners. You may remember from Chapter 2 that stress, unhappy events, loss, and numerous other circumstances can easily turn our vulnerability to depression into a reality. Now it's time to make sure that these bends in the road don't send you spinning. Using tried-and-true methods and some cutting-edge cognitive psychology, we'll give you the tools you need to stay depression-free. These are the same ones I use in my practice, and are similar to the methods used by psychologists all around the country. Depression-proofing your life—giving your mind the proper stimulation, socialization, and satisfaction—is as powerful as *any* medicine.

At the beginning of this book, I spoke of depression treatment as a four-legged chair; each leg had to be both sturdy and equal to the others for the chair to be stable. These four steps are the four legs, and the next few chapters will teach you how to build them. Cut one short, however, and the whole thing can wobble uneasily or even collapse.

6

How to Take SAM-e

Step 1—The Self-Assessment Test

Before you begin Step 2 (see page 122), we urge you to take a simple self-assessment test, the Depression Severity Scale. It will help determine whether you are truly suffering from depression, the degree of your depression, and the best way for you to take SAM-e. The test consists of only ten questions, but it can speak volumes about your mental state.

The Depression Severity Scale will also alert readers who are seriously depressed and should seek medical attention before self-treating their depression. This test was originally designed to give primary care doctors an easy yet reliable method to screen for depression during routine patient visits. It is easy enough for non-doctors to use, but sophisticated enough to differentiate between the different grades of depression, ranging from mild to moderate to severe. We don't want to suggest that using the Depression Severity Scale on your own is as good as getting a diagnosis from an experienced physician. Not at all. It is, however, a useful tool to help you sort out your symptoms and track your progress. By periodically retaking the test, you can measure your improvement over the next few weeks after you start taking SAM-e.

(Although we strongly urge people who are severely depressed to seek psychiatric intervention, we do not want to suggest that psychological counseling is useful only for the most severely depressed. Regardless of the degree of depression, many people can greatly benefit from some form of therapy—either individual or group—as well as from taking SAM-e.)

Now answer the questions on the Depression Severity Scale. When you are finished, tally up your score for the first nine questions. As you will see, the tenth is answered a bit differently. When you are done, we will explain how to interpret the results.

DEPRESSION SEVERITY SCALE

Over the last two weeks, how often have you been bothered by any of the following problems?

		Not at all	Several days	More than half the days	Nearly every day
1.	Little interest or pleasure in doing things	0	1	2	3
2.	Feeling down, depressed, or hopeless	0	1	2	3
3.	Trouble falling or staying asleep, or sleeping too much	0	1	2	3
4.	Feeling tired or having little energy	0	1	2	3
5.	Poor appetite or overeating	0	1	2	3
6.	Feeling bad about yourself—or that you are a failure or have let yourself or your family down	0	1	2	3

7. Trouble concentrat-
ing on things, such
as reading the news-
paper or watching
television   0   1   2   3

8. Moving or speaking
so slowly that other
people could have
noticed. Or the op-
posite—being so
fidgety or restless
that you have been
moving around a
lot more than usual   0   1   2   3

9. Thoughts that you
would be better off
dead, or of hurting
yourself in some
way   0   1   2   3

10. If you checked off *any* problems, how *difficult* have these problems made it for you to do your work, take care of things at home, or get along with other people?

Not difficult at all	Somewhat difficult	Very difficult	Extremely difficult
☐	☐	☐	☐

Adapted from the PRIME-MD Patient Health Question-naire®, developed by Drs. Robert L. Spitzer, Janet B.W.

*Williams, Kurt Kroenke, and colleagues. For research infor-
mation, contact Dr. Spitzer at rls8@columbia.edu. PRIME-
MD® is a trademark of Pfizer Inc. Copyright © 1999
Pfizer Inc. All rights reserved. Reproduced with permission.*

UNDERSTANDING THE RESULTS
OF THE DEPRESSION SEVERITY SCALE

IF YOU SCORED BETWEEN 0 AND 5: A score under 6 does not fall within the range of depression, with one important exception. If you answered yes to question 9, you should seek professional help. No thoughts of suicide should be dismissed. They could be an indication of a serious, life-threatening depression.

In most cases, however, a score of 0–5 is not depression. Although you may have an occasional bad mood, bad thought, or even bad day, you are not actually depressed.

This raises question: What if you did not officially fall into the depressed category, yet believe that you are indeed depressed? Maybe depression isn't your primary problem. There are many physical and psychological conditions that can resemble depression, and produce similar symptoms. (For more information, we refer you back to page 39.) If you are convinced, regardless of your test score, that you are depressed, we recommend that you get an evaluation from a qualified professional.

What if you scored 5 or below, yet your spouse, close relatives, or friends are telling you that you are depressed and are urging you to see a doctor? Listen to them! Self-assessment tests are notoriously poor for diagnosing severe depression, because people who are severely depressed often do not recognize their symptoms. Their behavior may seem "off" to others, but they are unaware of it. In fact, they don't even think there's anything wrong. The bottom line is, if everyone is telling you that you are depressed, but you don't agree—don't ignore it. See a doctor for a professional evaluation.

IF YOU SCORED BETWEEN 6 AND 12: This score suggests that you are in the gray zone, a low-level depression. Some of you may *always* feel somewhat low. Although you are able to function at work or at home, you may not be getting much joy out of life. Some of you may suffer from an episodic or mild depression that ebbs and rises. You may not feel bad all the time, yet your periodic depressions could still have a decidedly negative effect on your life. Until recently, gray zone depressions have not been considered serious enough to treat. We now know that they are often the prelude to more severe depressive episodes down the road and should be treated.

IF YOU SCORED BETWEEN 13 AND 18: This score suggests that you may suffer from mild-to-moderate depression. Some things to consider are: Is this your first depressive episode? Have you experienced similar periods of depression in the past? Have you experienced a low-level, or gray zone, depression before this more intense episode? These questions are important in helping to determine the right dose of SAM-e as well as the length of treatment, as I will explain later.

IF YOU SCORED BETWEEN 19 AND 27: This score suggests a more severe depression for which we do not recommend self-treatment. For best results, you should get an evaluation from a qualified physician, who will then monitor your treatment. SAM-e may still work well for you, either alone or in combination with other antidepressants. If your doctor is unfamiliar with SAM-e, show him or her this book. It will provide the information he or she needs to learn to use SAM-e effectively.

QUESTION 10: This last question measures functional impairment—that is, it helps to determine the impact your symptoms may be having on your life. If you checked off "Very difficult" or "Extremely difficult," you should get a medical evaluation before taking SAM-e. It takes a lot of courage to admit to yourself that you are being overwhelmed by your problems. Take heart in knowing that studies have shown that the sooner you get appropriate treatment, the better your chances for a quick and full recovery.

HOW TO USE THESE TESTS

As mentioned, the Depression Severity Scale will also help you to track your progress. Retake the test after your first two weeks on SAM-e. Not only should you be feeling better, but this should be reflected in an improvement of at least twenty-five percent on your score. So, if your initial score was 16, a twenty-five percent improvement would bring you down to 12. By week four, you should see an improvement of fifty percent. Retake the test after two more weeks to track your progress. You are in complete remission when your score is 5 or under. For most people, this should take no longer than six weeks.

Step 2—Everything You Need to Know About Taking SAM-e

WHAT IS THE RIGHT DOSE?

The starting dose of SAM-e is 400mg daily. This dose is usually effective for people with mild-to-moderate depression. Since SAM-e works quickly, most of you will probably see a significant improvement (of at least twenty-five percent) within two weeks. If you do not see a twenty-five percent improvement after two weeks, increase your dose of SAM-e to 800mg daily. After increasing your dose, retake the self-assessment test after two more weeks. If you still do not see a twenty-five percent improvement, we recommend that you seek a professional evaluation. You may need to take a higher dose of SAM-e to get a good response, or SAM-e in combination with another antidepressant, or a different antidepressant altogether. Caution: If you have a history of extreme sensitivity to medication, start out with a lower dose of 200mg daily for the first week. If you do not experience any problems, you can increase your dose to 400mg daily.

How do I know that SAM-e will work for me?

When you begin antidepressant therapy, it is important to understand that no antidepressant works one hundred percent of the time for everybody. Studies show that SAM-e is effective for seventy percent of the people who try it, which makes it is equal to—if not better than—other antidepressants. The odds are that SAM-e will lift you out of your depression, as it has the hundreds of thousands of people who are already using it successfully. If SAM-e doesn't work for you, however, don't get discouraged. It doesn't mean that you have failed or that there is anything wrong with you. All it means is that you may respond better to a different antidepressant, or need to add another antidepressant to your regimen. As you know, SAM-e can be used very effectively along with other antidepressants to speed up and improve a patient's response, or to lower the dose of prescription antidepressants to minimize side effects.

Where can I buy SAM-e?

Gone are the days when we had to special-order SAM-e from a pharmacy in Italy and pray that it arrived in time for our patients! Today, you can buy SAM-e at major chain stores, including pharmacies; at health food stores, and at mass merchandisers such as grocery stores, drugstores, and discount stores.

How is SAM-e sold?

SAM-e is sold in tablet form, either packaged in an airtight blister pack or sold loose in a plastic bottle. Be sure to buy enteric-coated SAM-e. This preparation is the most stable and best absorbed by the body. Enteric-coated SAM-e is very stable and stays effective for up to five years as long as it is not exposed to moisture. If the tablets get moist, be sure to use them up within a month or they may lose their potency. To be on the safe side, keep your SAM-e in a closed bottle or blister pack until you are ready to use it. Store it in a dry place like your kitchen cabinet. Do not store SAM-e in the refrigerator, because it could pick up moisture.

When is the best time to take SAM-e?

To maximize its effectiveness, SAM-e should be taken on an empty stomach about half an hour before meals. Tailor the time you take your dose to best suit your needs. If you are taking 400mg of SAM-e daily, you can either take the full amount in the morning, or take 200mg before breakfast and 200mg before lunch.

As noted in Chapter 5, some people find that the afternoon dose gives them a mild energy boost. If your energy is depleted in the afternoon, taking the second half of your SAM-e regimen in the afternoon may help. If you take 800mg of SAM-e daily, you should take 400mg before breakfast and 400mg before lunch. Rarely, some people may find that taking SAM-e on an empty stomach will cause heartburn. If this happens to you, try taking it with your meals.

How long should I take SAM-e?

There is absolutely no evidence that taking SAM-e long-term poses any risk to your health. In fact, as I have discussed, it does many good things for your body. The question of how long you take it depends on your progress. Although SAM-e works rapidly, it is wise not to discontinue your medication until you have experienced a *full* and *lasting* recovery. Why? If you are not fully recovered, you run a high risk of recurrence. If you have mild depression, we recommend taking SAM-e for a minimum of four months after you have achieved a fifty percent improvement on your self-assessment chart. Frankly, since SAM-e rarely causes any side effects and probably offers significant health benefits, we recommend staying on it longer, perhaps up to nine months. There's no harm in staying on SAM-e even longer if you want to.

If you have a history of more than three serious depressive episodes, you run a very high chance of a recurrence. Therefore, we recommend that you take

SAM-e indefinitely. This is particularly important for people who don't recognize when they are becoming depressed, and who may get profoundly depressed before they seek treatment. With each relapse, it is increasingly difficult to find an effective antidepressant. Thus, if SAM-e is working to keep you out of depression, stick with it.

What happens if I miss a dose (or even a day) of my SAM-e? Should I double up on my next dose?

If you miss your morning dose, you can take the entire dose before lunch. However, if you miss a day, don't try to make up for it the next. Rather, continue on your normal dose. Keep in mind that SAM-e cannot work unless you take it consistently. If you miss an occasional day, that's fine, but if you continually skip your dose, you run the risk of relapse. If you find that you are forgetting to take your SAM-e, devise a way of reminding yourself. Keep track of your daily doses on your calendar or keep a chart posted in an area at home or work where you are likely to see it.

Can I overdose on SAM-e?

No. SAM-e has been given in doses up to 3600mg daily with no adverse effects. There are no reports of death due to overdosing with SAM-e. However, at very high doses you may experience some gastrointestinal distress, including diarrhea and heartburn. Therefore, we recommend that you stick to our recommended doses.

Is SAM-e addictive? If I discontinue taking it, can I develop withdrawal symptoms as one does with other antidepressants?

No, SAM-e is not addictive. There are no reports of people developing any problems at all if they discontinue taking SAM-e, except of course, that they are at risk of relapsing back into depression. (Patients taking SRIs, however, should *never* discontinue their medication abruptly; rather, it should be gradually tapered off. If they do suddenly stop taking their medication, they could develop extremely unpleasant withdrawal symptoms that resemble the early stages of flu, right down to the headache and muscle ache. These symptoms can last for up to two weeks.)

Are there any side effects from SAM-e, however rare?

Studies have shown that patients develop fewer side effects on SAM-e than they do on placebos! Nevertheless, nothing—not even sugar pills—is completely side-effect-free. On rare occasions, people may develop a mild headache when they begin taking SAM-e, which usually disappears after the first week or two. At high doses (more than we recommend) SAM-e can cause diarrhea. What you don't see with SAM-e are the weight gain, sexual dysfunction, anxiety attacks, and chronic gastrointestinal distress that are side effects of other antidepressants. (As noted earlier, SAM-e should not be taken by patients with bipolar depression unless they are under the supervision of a psychiatrist knowledgeable in mood disorder treatment. Like other antidepressants, SAM-e can induce a manic phase in bipolar patients.)

Can I drink alcoholic beverages while taking SAM-e?

Although we usually advise people who are taking antidepressants not to drink, there is no reason to abstain when you are taking SAM-e. Alcohol does not adversely affect SAM-e in any way. But remember that alcohol is a depressant, and should not be used by people who have not fully recovered from their depression. Nor should alcohol ever be used by people who have a problem with alcohol dependency. Since SAM-e has a beneficial effect on liver function, it is an excellent antidepressant for recovering alcoholics. It has also been used, along with other prescription and nonprescription drugs, to help relieve alcohol dependency. In fact, one Italian study showed that SAM-e made it easier for people addicted to alcohol and painkillers to quit. Many people who suffer from substance abuse find that when they start taking SAM-e, they no longer have a strong craving for alcohol or other drugs.

Are there any medications that have harmful interactions with SAM-e?

SAM-e is unique among antidepressants in that no adverse effects have ever been reported when it is taken with other medications. This includes drugs used to treat heart conditions and high blood pressure, when antidepressants are normally contraindicated. While

SAM-e is generally safe when combined with other drugs, there may be one exception: MAO inhibitors. Although it has never been studied, given the fact that MAO inhibitors interact poorly with so many other drugs, do not combine them with SAM-e. If you are taking other medication, it is wise to tell your physician that you are also taking SAM-e.

I think that my child is depressed. Is it safe to give him SAM-e?

If you think your child is depressed, you must have him evaluated by a qualified physician. Depression in children is very difficult to diagnose and can often be caused by problems such as substance abuse, medical conditions, or even poor family relationships. SAM-e may be a good choice for your child, but you must first seek the appropriate medical attention so that you can get an accurate diagnosis.

Can SAM-e be taken with St. John's wort?

There's no reason why not. We sometimes prescribe SAM-e with St. John's wort for people who have not fully responded to either antidepressant alone.

Should I take any other nutritional supplements with SAM-e?

We recommend that you take 800mcg of folate (folic acid) and 1000mcg (1mg) of vitamin B_{12} daily. These vitamins are required for making the amino acid methionine, essential for SAM-e production in the body. Terry's studies have shown that at least one third of all depressed patients are folate-deficient, which can hamper their recovery. In fact, people who take folate along with an antidepressant recover better and faster than those who don't, whether or not they have low folate levels. (For more information, turn to Chapter 7, "The Stop Depression Now Food Plan.") You can take SAM-e with any other vitamins, minerals, or supplements you may be taking.

I'm a nursing mother suffering from the postpartum blues. Is it safe for my infant if I take SAM-e?

There is no easy way to answer this question; all we can do is give you the facts. SAM-e has been given to pregnant women for short periods at high doses (1600mg daily) with no reported adverse effects on either mother or child. Levels of SAM-e are naturally quite high in newborns, so it reasonable to assume that it is safe for infants if it passes through the breast milk. Nevertheless, any drug you take while you are nursing requires careful consideration. Although SAM-e is probably safe, we can't say that it or any other antidepressant is absolutely one hundred percent, guaranteed safe for newborns. There are simply no long-term studies. If you are so despondent that you cannot function, or are so despondent that you are worried that you may physically abuse your child, you will probably need to take some antidepressant. Before you self-medicate, however, you should be evaluated by a physician. About sixty percent of all cases of severe postpartum depression would fall into the bipolar category, in which cases SAM-e would not be the appropriate choice.

I have seasonal affective disorder (SAD). Should I take SAM-e every day?

Although there are no controlled studies on the use of SAM-e for SAD, we have clinical experience using it successfully with SAD patients. Many of these patients also benefit from additional light therapy. As to how to take SAM-e, it all depends on the type of SAD you are experiencing. Many people who suffer from SAD become extremely active in the summer. They are full of excess energy, sleep less than they do in the fall and winter, and often appear to be in overdrive. If this sounds like you, then you should only take SAM-e from October through April. If you take it in the summer, it could make you manic. If, on the other hand, your mood is down at any time of the year but usually worsens in winter, then you may benefit from taking SAM-e all year round.

If I'm having difficulty sleeping, what natural supplements can I use with SAM-e?

Sleep disturbances are quite common during depression, and taking a sleep aid, whether it's prescription or natural, can be very helpful. My favorite natural sleep remedy is a mix of the hormone melatonin, lemon balm, and passionflower; it works well for many of my patients. I do not recommend the herb valerian because it can sometimes leave a hangover in the morning. For some people, an over-the-counter antihistamine can do the trick. If over-the-counter remedies do not work, then talk to your doctor about prescription medication.

But remember, getting a good night's sleep involves more than popping a pill. I try to teach my patients good sleep hygiene. Going to sleep at around the same time every night and getting up around the same time every morning can help restore the body's natural sleep rhythm. Getting proper exercise during the day can have an amazing effect on the quality of sleep at night. Learn to relax and "de-stress" before bedtime. For some tips on how to unwind, see Chapter 8 ("A Simple Guide to Depression-Proofing Your Life").

7

The Stop Depression
Now Food Plan

SAM-e can restore balance to your brain chemistry, but it doesn't provide the one thing that your brain cells need to stay healthy—good nutrition. Although most of us know that diet can help prevent *physical* diseases such as osteoporosis, cancer, and heart disease, we don't think that food can strengthen our *mental* health. Yet what we eat can have an equally profound impact on our emotional state. Yes, you can eat to beat depression.

For nearly two decades, much of Terry's research has focused on the role of nutrition in the treatment and prevention of depression. From Terry's research we know that the levels of key nutrients are often low in depressed people. Poor nutrition can aggravate an existing depression, but in some cases, nutritional deficiencies themselves may be *triggers* for depression. Closing the nutritional gap is an important step in healing depression. This chapter will reinforce the power of good nutrition and show how simple but smart changes in your diet can make an enormous difference in how you feel.

Food provides not only the fuel for living but also the basic components for the maintenance and repair of cells *all* over the body . . . including the brain. The Stop Depression Now food plan can enhance the effect of SAM-e by giving your cells the nutrients they need to maintain optimal health. The beauty of our food plan is that it works not only for the brain but for everywhere else in the body too.

When food enters your mouth, a complex process begins that can build toward a healthy brain and mind. But there are substances in our foods that can help us and others that can harm us. The key is achieving the right balance.

Many of us are out of balance. We eat too much of the wrong foods and not enough of the right ones. Modern food-processing techniques, combined with our hectic lifestyles, leave us with a diet stripped of many important nutrients—a detriment to our mental and physical health. Deficiencies in key vitamins (particularly B vitamins) and minerals can trigger or aggravate depression. Read this chapter carefully to make sure that you are getting enough of the nutrients necessary to maintain your well-being.

By the way, eating should not be a chore! Mealtime should be a relaxing, pleasant experience, a time to relieve stress. Don't force yourself to eat foods that you hate, in the name of good health. With all the variety among the foods we recommend, you can surely find at least some that are pleasing to your palate.

The Basics

Before we get specific, here are some general guidelines. As many of you know, there are three basic types of nutrients: proteins, carbohydrates, and fats. A balanced diet consists of the right type of each of these nutrients in the right amount.

Carbohydrates, found in vegetables, fruits, cereals, grains, and legumes, are a strong source of energy. Between forty and fifty percent of daily food intake should be some form of carbohydrate. Essentially there are two kinds of carbohydrates—simple and complex. The good carbohydrates are complex. These are fruits and vegetables, whole-grain unrefined products such as multigrain breads and cereals, and pasta made from whole-wheat or vegetable flours. They break down slowly in the body, and do not cause a sharp rise in blood sugar. The bad carbohydrates (simple carbohydrates) are found in refined flour, cakes, cookies, soda, chips, and other foods with high sugar content. They tend to cause a sharper rise in blood sugar. Eating too many bad carbohydrates can result in a sugar crash, leaving you hungry, depleted, and feeling down. Although it's never been studied, we believe that a high-sugar diet may contribute to depression by creating sugar "highs and lows" that can result in sagging spirits. Sticking to complex carbohydrates—and avoiding junk food—can help keep you off the sugar roller coaster. Ideally, you should limit your servings of white bread, cereal, or pasta to no more than four a day. (One serving is equal to one slice of bread, or one cup of rice or pasta.)

Proteins are found in all meat (including poultry and fish), dairy products, and plant foods such as beans. Protein is essential to building, maintaining, and repairing body tissue. It helps to reduce the effects of fast-burning carbohydrates. Twenty to thirty percent of your daily food intake should be in some form of protein.

And yes, you need *fats!* Between twenty and thirty percent of your daily calories should be in some form of fat. Fat is essential for the production and maintenance of cell membranes and the formation of hormones, and is required for other important jobs in the body. In fact, eating the right kind of fat may be key to preventing depression, as we'll discuss later.

These three nutrients form the building blocks of a depression-proof diet, but within each category, there are many variables. As you will see, it all comes down to making the right food choices.

Controlling Homocysteine

Eating the right foods, and taking the right supplements, can help control an important risk factor for depression—elevated homocysteine levels. In Chapter 3, we stressed the importance of preventing excessive levels of homocysteine, an amino acid produced by our cells which in high amounts can be very dangerous. Now we're going to tell you exactly what you need to do to control this potential troublemaker.

At normal levels, homocysteine is not bad. In fact, it is part of the chemical pathway in the body that produces two very important chemicals: methionine, the amino acid that becomes SAM-e, and glutathione, the body's primary antioxidant. As you may remember, SAM-e is involved in the process of converting homocysteine to methionine and later to glutathione. When the body is working well, homocysteine is put to good use.

When things go wrong and homocysteine is allowed to accumulate, it can cause a great deal of destruction. High levels of homocysteine (over 14mcg/liter) have been linked to an increased risk of heart disease, stroke, different types of cancer, Alzheimer's disease, and depression. Homocysteine levels tend to rise with age, and so does the risk of developing many different mental and physical ailments. But homocysteine can cause trouble at any age.

In a recent study of patients with dementia and other psychiatric disorders, including major depression, the homocysteine levels in their blood were found to be significantly elevated as compared with those of people in good mental health. The same is true for patients suffering from chronic fatigue syndrome.

The body has its own built-in system to control homocysteine. It involves the methylation cycle (described in Chapter 3), which is the process by which homocysteine is converted into methionine and SAM-e. The methylation cycle is dependent on two key B vitamins: folate (also known as folic acid) and vitamin B_{12}. Unfortunately, because of poor dietary habits, many of us may become deficient in these B vitamins. To make matters worse, methylation declines with age, allowing homocysteine to rise.

There is a great deal you can do to control homocysteine on your own. First, moderate elevations of homocysteine may often result from lifestyle factors that can easily be modified. These are smoking, a high level of coffee consumption, and too little physical exercise. Aside from these adjustments to your lifestyle, there are some other things you can do.

EAT MORE FOLATE. As noted above, folate is a B vitamin that boosts the methylation cycle, thereby lowering homocysteine levels. Along with vitamin B_{12}, it is essential for the formation of methionine, the building block of SAM-e. Low serum folate levels are associated with an increased risk of depression, as is a deficiency in SAM-e. In a review article coauthored by Terry on the health effects of homocysteine, mentioned in Chapter 6, he reported that up to thirty percent of all people suffering from depression are also folate-deficient. Folate deficiency may be as high as ninety percent in elderly populations with psychiatric disorders, including depression and dementia. In another study coauthored by Terry and Maurizio Fava at the Harvard-affiliated Massachusetts General Hospital, they reported that in a group of 213 depressed patients, about one third had abnormally low levels of either folate or B_{12}, or elevated serum homocysteine levels. They also noted that patients who were folate-deficient were less likely to respond to treatment with Prozac. This falls in line with another study that Terry coauthored and published in the medical journal *The Lancet.* There Terry and his colleagues showed that depressed patients receiving standard prescription antidepressants had a significantly better clinical outcome when supplemented with folate. As you can see, folate is essential for the maintenance of mood and a full response to antidepressant treatment.

Derived from the same root as the word *foliage,* folate is found in dark green leafy vegetables (such as spinach and broccoli), dried beans, bananas, orange juice, yeast, peanuts, sunflower seeds, wheat germ, and fortified breakfast cereals.

Obviously, we should all strive to include more folate-rich foods in our diets. To preserve folate content in foods such as legumes or vegetables, don't overcook! Lightly steam or sauté your vegetables so that they are still firm. Eat whole-grain unprocessed breads and cereals. These healthy foods not only boost folate but also protect against many different diseases, from heart disease to cancer to diabetes. To be on the safe side, since so many of us eat erratically and because folate is volatile, we recommend taking a folate supplement of 800mcg daily. We feel the RDA of 400mcg daily is inadequate; 800mcg is needed to protect against elevated homocysteine and to reduce the risk of heart attacks, strokes, and birth defects.

WATCH YOUR B_{12} LEVELS. Although it has received less attention than folate, B_{12} is also instrumental in controlling homocysteine. While B_{12} deficiency is quite common among older people, it can hamper mental performance at any age. B_{12} assists folate in the production of methionine, as well as in regulating the formation of red blood cells. It also helps in the utilization of iron, which is required for proper digestion and absorption of foods. B_{12} is found in red meat, poultry, fish, eggs, and dairy products. With the exception of fish, these are foods that many people have cut down on to reduce their intake of saturated fat. Although fish is healthy, as we will discuss later, Americans don't eat enough of it. Lean cuts of meat and low-fat dairy products are a good source of B_{12} and can be included in a healthy diet. And despite popular belief, there is no evidence that eggs promote high cholesterol levels. They can be eaten in moderation.

Even if you eat the right foods, you may not get

enough B_{12}. As with folate, microwave cooking can destroy as much as half of the B_{12} content in food. If you're over sixty-five, the odds of developing a deficiency are high, due to poor absorption of B_{12}. At least ten percent of the elderly population is B_{12}-deficient. B_{12} deficiency can cause severe neurological symptoms, including balance problems, tingling in the hands and feet, memory loss, dementia, and depression. In fact, if older people exhibit any of these symptoms, they should have their B_{12} levels checked. B_{12} supplementation can reverse many of the symptoms, either alone or with other treatments. Remember, as we age, our homocysteine levels are rising. At the same time, our stomachs produce less of the hydrochloric acid critical to the absorption of B_{12}.

The solution is to take B_{12} supplements. We recommend 1000mcg (1mg) daily for everyone regardless of age, especially if you are taking a folate supplement. Folate can mask the symptoms of B_{12} deficiency, making it difficult to diagnose. In order to prevent any problem, take B_{12} along with your folate.

OTHER IMPORTANT B VITAMINS. Low levels of vitamin B_1 (thiamine) and vitamin B_6 can also increase the risk of depression. Unrefined whole-grain cereals or fortified cereals are an excellent source of these B vitamins. Thiamine in particular can be destroyed by alcohol, so excessive drinkers are at great risk of a deficiency in this vitamin. If you take a multivitamin, as many people do, you will probably get enough of these B vitamins to prevent a deficiency.

B vitamins are not the whole story. If you're going to eat to beat depression, you're going to need more of something that many of you have cut back on: fat.

Why Fat Is Good

People who are seeking to shed pounds often follow low-fat diets. On the surface this makes sense, because each gram of fat has twice the calories of an equivalent amount of protein or carbohydrate. If you cut out fat, you might assume that you would produce more lean tissue (muscle).

Ironically, though, diets that are restricted in fats can actually cause you to *gain* fat and *lose* muscle. First, our bodies don't function at optimum levels without some fat; it is necessary for the production of hormones and the absorption of fat-soluble vitamins. Second, if you don't eat some fat with your carbohydrates you are likely to get hungrier faster, and consequently, you'll overeat. Carbohydrates trigger the release of insulin, sending sugar into muscle cells. The excess of this sugar is stored as fat. But eating a small amount of fat along with carbohydrates can slow down this process, giving your body time to burn the extra calories before they are converted to fat.

Essential fatty acids, however, are an entirely different matter . . . and unfortunately, in this country, are largely underconsumed and misunderstood. For instance, these fats protect against heart disease and can actually lower cholesterol.

And they can play a key role in depression.

Essential Fatty Acids

Essential fatty acids (EFAs) are polyunsaturated fatty acids that cannot be produced by the human body and must therefore be obtained from diet. As the structural components of membranes, EFAs help form a barrier that keeps foreign molecules, viruses, yeasts, fungi, and bacteria outside of cells, and retains proteins, enzymes, and genetic material inside. Changes in fatty acid intake may modify cell membrane fluidity, affecting receptors, membrane-based enzymes, permeability, and neurotransmitter transport. These critical functions at the cellular level have a lot to do with brain activity and underline the importance of EFAs in depression. Recent studies have linked a diet low in omega-3 fatty acids to a higher incidence of depression, aggression, dementia, and ADHD (attention deficit disorder with hyperactivity).

There are two types of essential fatty acids: omega-

6 and omega-3. Most people get adequate amounts of omega-6 fatty acids through their diet but not nearly enough omega-3.

Omega-6 fatty acids are found in nuts, seeds, avocados, grains, and most cooking oils. Omega-3 fatty acids are generally found in cold-water fatty fish, deep green vegetables, and some grains and seeds. Our hunter-gatherer ancestors had a ratio of omega-6 to omega-3 fatty acids of about 5:1. Our modern food processing and changes in diet have adjusted that ratio to 24:1. It is critical to your health to turn back the clock on this imbalance.

OMEGA-3 AND DHA

Omega-3 fatty acids contain alpha-linolenic acid, which in turn is metabolized into eicosapentaenoic acid (EPA) and docosahexaenoic acid (DHA) in the body. Found in high concentrations in the gray matter of the brain and the retina of the eye, DHA is the building block of human brain tissue. As we discussed in Chapter 3, the brain's gray matter is composed of billions of cells. Each cell signals electrochemically to its counterparts through the synapses, and adequate amounts of DHA ensure that this process runs smoothly. Deficiencies in omega-3 fatty acids such as DHA may contribute to depression, impaired brain function, and heart disease.

Over the past fifty years the consumption of omega-3 fatty acids has significantly declined in the West. We are ingesting less DHA and instead eating more omega-6 fatty acids. Not only have we reduced our intake of fish, but we are not eating as many of the whole grains and seeds filled with omega-3 fatty acids.

Studies have shown that people who live near coastal regions where fresh fish is abundant are the happiest, and people who live inland where fresh fish is not as easy to find are the most depressed. In an article published in 1995 in the *American Journal of Clinical Nutrition,* authors Dr. Joseph R. Hibbeln and Dr. Norman Salem, Jr., of the National Institutes of Health noted the documented increase in depression in North America during this last century, a period in which the consumption of DHA declined. While recognizing that the "many stresses of modern life contribute" to the prevalence of depression, they add that "relative deficiencies in omega-3 essential fatty acids (such as DHA) may also intensify vulnerability to depression."

Good sources of DHA are foods that many people have given up in the name of good health, such as organ meats (which are high in saturated fat and toxins) and eggs. But DHA is also abundant in fatty fish like salmon, mackerel, sardines, flounder, and albacore tuna. It is essential to consume two to three servings of fish per week to maintain proper levels of DHA. Recently scientists have developed techniques to extract DHA from the microalgae these fish ingest, and DHA supplements are now available.

FLAXSEED OIL: A KEY OMEGA-3 SOURCE

Thousands of years ago, our hunter-gatherer ancestors ate flax along with other wild grasses. Although they were unaware of its benefits, flaxseed contains more omega-3 than fatty fish. (It is not yet clear if flaxseed oil has the same benefit for the heart as fish oil. Further research is needed.)

The downside is that flax is not easy to use. It is notoriously unstable and unless properly processed can turn rancid very quickly. Fresh flaxseed can also be purchased at health food stores and ground up in a coffee grinder for a smoother consistency. Sprinkle about a quarter of a cup of fresh-ground flaxseed on hot or cold cereal for a wonderful supplement of omega-3 fatty acid. Flaxseed cold cereals are also available at health food stores. They are actually quite delicious!

Some people may find omega-3 sources such as fish and flaxseed oils hard on the digestive system, even though there is evidence that they are helpful in inflammatory bowel disease. For these people, perilla oil is an alternative.

The Right Minerals

Minerals are naturally occurring chemical elements found throughout the human body: in the bones, muscles, teeth, blood, and—of special relevance to this book—nerve cells. Deficiencies in two key minerals can contribute to mood disorders.

MAGNESIUM. Magnesium is a hardworking mineral that we too often take for granted. It is involved in nearly every essential bodily function, from the maintenance of the heart muscle to the creation of bone and the regulation of blood sugar. It is so important that it is called the "gatekeeper" of cellular activity. Magnesium deficiency can also cause numerous psychological changes, including depression. This is borne out in research. Plasma magnesium levels have been found to be significantly lower in depressed patients than in controls. The symptoms of magnesium deficiency include poor attention, memory loss, fear, restlessness, insomnia, muscle cramps, and dizziness. Foods rich in magnesium include wheat bran, whole grains, leafy green vegetables, low-fat dairy products, lean cuts of meat, beans, bananas, apricots, dry mustard, curry powder, and cocoa. Surely there's something on this list that you like!

CALCIUM. Your body needs calcium to complete the magnesium picture. These two minerals work well in tandem. Good food sources of calcium are low-fat dairy products, fortified breakfast cereals, salmon and sardines with bones, tofu (if made with calcium sulfate), and blackstrap molasses. It may surprise you to learn that most women do not have adequate calcium intake at any age. In fact, a recent study showed that 1200mg of calcium a day helped PMS symptoms.

Antioxidant-Rich Foods

In Chapter 3, we discussed how SAM-e boosts levels of glutathione, an important antioxidant produced by every cell in the body. As we pointed out, antioxidants are important because they protect us against free radicals, chemicals produced in the body which can injure healthy cells and tissues. Scientists now believe that free radicals are a major factor in nearly every known disease—including heart disease, arthritis, Alzheimer's disease, Parkinson's disease, and perhaps even depression. Your brain is particularly vulnerable to free radical damage for two reasons. First, it is a hotbed of activity. Brain cells need a constant flow of blood and oxygen to produce energy. This increases the production of free radicals. Second, more than fifty percent of the brain is composed of fat, making it vulnerable to lipid peroxidation and the formation of free radicals.

If free radicals start to destroy brain cells, they wreak havoc with neurotransmitters, destroying membranes and receptors. Many researchers suspect that free radical damage to neurons may inhibit the ability of nerve cells to produce adequate levels of neurotransmitters and other chemicals in the brain that organize thought and help cells communicate. This can create a chemical imbalance in the brain, and a cascade of problems such as depression, panic disorder, and anxiety attacks. Scientists believe that replenishing antioxidants through foods and supplements will help your brain retain its health and keep your mental edge sharp. Although the body produces some antioxidants on its own, we don't make enough to protect ourselves against free radicals.

Try to incorporate at least some of these foods into your daily diet.

FRESH VEGETABLES AND GREENS. You need to eat a full assortment of different types of vegetables to get full antioxidant protection. Deep green leafy vegetables such as spinach and kale have phytochemicals and antioxidants that are different from those of orange and yellow fruits and vegetables such as cantaloupe and winter squash. Cruciferous vegetables, such as broccoli, cauliflower, brussels sprouts, and cabbage, are good sources of antioxidants as well as other cancer-fighting phytochemicals.

All greens contain antioxidant flavonoids. They are loaded with minerals such as calcium and vitamins C and E. Look for beet greens, watercress, collard greens, mustard greens, and Swiss chard, which are excellent sources of antioxidants. Eat spinach! It not only contains antioxidants but is also a great source of folic acid. Interestingly, greens are powerful protectors against the most common cause of blindness—macular degeneration.

It would be ideal to eat five to eight half-cup servings of different vegetables every day.

FRESH FRUITS. Apples, berries, oranges, melons, grapes—all of nature's delicious bounty: fresh fruits are a wonderful source of natural antioxidants. Just to prove that something good for you doesn't have to taste lousy, a recent study showed that blueberries are number one in proanthocyanidins—the most potent of the dietary antioxidants.

DRIED FRUITS. Dried apricots and peaches are terrific sources of beta carotene, a natural antioxidant.

GARLIC AND ONIONS. These belong to the allium family, which also includes leeks and chives, and are a rich source of antioxidants.

RED GRAPES AND WINE. Red grapes and wine are excellent sources of antioxidants. A glass of red wine daily is good for your health, but should be avoided if you have a problem with alcohol dependency or are taking a medication that will interact poorly with alcohol. Some people find that alcohol can trigger their depression. If you are alcohol-sensitive, avoid it. As a substitute, consider grape leaves and peanuts.

SOY. The Japanese have a much longer life span than the people of any other nation with the exception of Ireland. Traditional Japanese cuisine is rich in food derived from soy, including tofu, bean curd, tempeh (fermented soybean patty), miso (fermented bean paste), and edamame (roasted soybeans). Soybeans contain many disease-fighting phytochemicals that are simply not found in foods consumed in the West.

TEA. All types of tea contain antioxidant flavonoids called polyphenols which are also present in red wine. The polyphenols in green tea may be more potent than those found in other teas.

Stop!

I think it's always a good idea to have a clear picture of what you shouldn't eat, so I'm going to lay it out for you plain and simple. Your cells depend on it!

- Don't eat processed meat. Saturated fat and chemicals such as nitrates are converted in the stomach into potentially carcinogenic chemicals called nitrosamines. Nitrosamines promote the formation of free radicals.

- Don't eat "bad fats." Most of us know that it is wise to cut down on saturated fat, which can raise blood cholesterol levels, but you should also avoid hydrogenated fats (such as margarine) or partially hydrogenated fats. These fats can promote the formation of transfatty acids in the body, which raise blood cholesterol levels and increase the risk of breast cancer. Become an alert consumer! You won't know whether a food contains hydrogenated or partially hydrogenated fat unless you read the label.

- Don't eat white bread, sugared breakfast foods, snack and junk foods! Replace with whole-grain breads, rye, or pumpernickel.
- Remember, don't indulge in classic vices. Smoking, a low nutritional intake of vitamins, and high coffee consumption, along with too little physical exercise, can raise levels of homocysteine. So can excessive alcohol.

The right food can help promote the conditions in your body that enhance your physical and mental health. It will give your body the raw materials it needs to maintain mood, strength, and stamina.

In Chapter 8, you will learn about the fourth and last component of the Stop Depression Now program—how to depression-proof your life.

8

A Simple Guide to Depression-Proofing Your Life

SAM-e combined with the Stop Depression Now food plan will lift you out of your depression and bring you back to life. In order to *stay* depression-free, however, you will also need to make some positive changes in your lifestyle.

The Stop Depression Now program has four dimensions that will transport you from depression to well-being. The first three steps in the program help restore the normal balance between neurotransmitters. They deal with the biology of depression. Step 4, however, will help you better cope with the external factors that may be contributing to or even triggering your depression. To underscore the importance of this piece of the program, I use the analogy of a car after a tune-up. Its tires are rotated, its chrome is sparkling clean, and it's ready for action. Put the key in the ignition and it purrs like a kitten. Yet if you drive recklessly and take life's curves the wrong way, you can still spin out of control. This chapter gives you the skills you need to help you stay firmly planted on the road to recovery—no matter how twisty it is.

Learning these skills is especially important because relapse is common with people who suffer from depression. Learning how to handle the stress that leads to depression can keep an episode from getting out of control, and perhaps even stave it off altogether. The techniques that I describe below are simple, yet these basic changes in your lifestyle and outlook can have a powerful effect.

One Step at a Time

Conquering even the mildest of depressions is often perceived as a daunting task—too weighty and complex to be undertaken. Poor self-esteem, destructive behaviors, and an overactive stress response all contribute to the sense that the depression is insurmountable—and that it would take Herculean strength to change it. Sufferers desperately want to turn these feelings off, but lacking the energy to do anything big enough to accomplish this task, they do nothing.

The good news is that there are things you can do to start whittling away at your depression, easily and without too much effort.

The first thing you must do is to *lower* your expectations. You can't change your behavior overnight. You need to view this process as one that moves along, one small step at a time. Instead of keeping your eye on the ultimate goal—which is feeling free of the fog you walk through, or the ton of bricks weighing on your chest—you need to be pleased if you can see clearly just a few feet farther ahead than you could before, and to feel satisfied that you can remove one brick at a time.

While that may not seem enough, consider this: Your small steps—baby steps, even—get you started on a long road. But this isn't like any other journey. With every step you take, no matter how small, the distance you still have to travel diminishes by far more than the ground you've covered. While each step might seem tiny, your stride grows every time you plant your foot. You'll be eating up the road to recovery in no time.

Here's how this plays out in real life. The dreaded company Christmas party is around the corner. This year, you are determined to push aside your depression and take part in the festivities. You imagine that you are going to move around the room chatting and trading repartee, and feel like the life of the party. But now it's hours before the occasion and already you feel completely overwhelmed and stressed out, convinced that your efforts will fail. Here's what you can learn from this experience:

- Clinging to a fantasy that is too big for your reality can cause you to freeze, making it highly unlikely that you will be able to attempt even a small change in the way you operate.

- Setting a smaller goal will ultimately feel more manageable both in anticipation and in reality. You won't sap yourself of the energy you desperately need to make small changes if you face only a step over a crack, rather than the paralyzing fear of a leap over a canyon.

- Smaller goals make it more likely that you'll be able to keep on improving. Each step doesn't seem too hard, but the distance you cover keeps growing. Looking back over how far you've traveled can boost your self-esteem and help you to realize just how much is in your power to accomplish. Success breeds success.

So, quite literally, what is a measured expectation? Before going to that corporate event, try writing down goals that seem doable:

"I will find one person, and in a quiet way (I do not have to be witty), I will discuss what's been going on at work, or even something about the event at hand."

"If I am seated at a table with people who seem to be ignoring me, I will listen closely to the conversation and strive to insert only an occasional comment. That will be enough."

"If I'm feeling desperately low and wishing I could

leave, I will complete one pleasant conversation before I go."

Instead of walking out of the party defeated, unhappy, and feeling like a failure, by simply achieving your small goals you can feel you have accomplished something.

Depressed people feel they have no control over their lives, but regulating your expectations puts you back into control by stacking the cards in your favor. Consider the challenge before you (the Christmas party). Place yourself in a context that's manageable (finding one person to chat with) and includes a simple step forward (completing a brief, pleasant conversation). Chances are, you will gain mastery over the moment.

You should think about expectations during every attempt you make to forestall or move past your depression. This factors into every aspect we will discuss in this chapter: social connections, exercise, relaxation techniques, pursuit of hobbies and other means of self-expression, and the management of what you will learn are your triggers for an episode of depression.

Know Your Triggers

It is not easy to head off or manage a depressive episode, but the odds of exerting a positive force over it increase if you know your triggers. You may not always be able to control when depression hits, or even the course it takes. But the more cognizant you are of its looming possibility, or sensitive to an event that could set it off, the easier it will be to move through the episode free of confusion, panic, and a sense of doom. "I'm feeling depressed because once again I felt belittled at the department meeting," is easier to address than, "I'm feeling worthless. Nothing I do seems to amount to anything." One thought has parameters. The other is a free-floating mass that can consume every constructive thought in its path. If you had a cold you'd take care of it so that it didn't blossom into pneumonia. The same principle applies to depression.

A good way to become familiar with your profile of triggers is to look separately at your work, social, and intimate life. Take a piece of paper and write down the names of people who in the past have set you off. Consider what it was they said or did and how it made you feel. Step back and consider the portrait, and ask yourself some key questions about these people and what they say and do:

- Do they criticize, or make sympathetic remarks that you read as pity?
- Is there a particular trait some people possess that leaves you feeling "less than"?
- Is there a circumstance that typically fills you with an unbearable envy?

The object is to become as clear as possible about the circumstances and interactions that trigger your depressions. This will not protect you from their appearance on the scene, but recognizing the triggers can give you a distance that helps contain the depression, just as a large object looks small from a distance. "Here comes Lily with that imperious look on her face. I'm sure there must have been a mistake in my report. This usually makes me crazy, but I'm going to simply correct the mistake and try to shut out her attitude."

You may of course get down on yourself as you proceed through the corrections, but that voice that says, "You always feel like this when you make a mistake," will help take the edge off the experience. "I'm hard on myself," you might even mutter silently to yourself with self-empathy—and that personal forgiveness is absolutely what you deserve.

By listing your triggers, you objectify them. They take on a shape and size you can manage. And in some instances, you might even be able to prepare. If walking into a party where you don't know anyone usually ends with your standing in the corner battling a depression, then come prepared. Check the newspaper before you leave the house so that you're able to bring up timely or interesting subjects. Ask your hostess in advance to tell you a bit about a few of her guests so you'll have some good questions in mind when introduced.

You can't rid yourself of a trigger, but you can control it before it controls you.

Look Again, Differently

Depression can easily lead to a distorted perception of the world, illogical thinking, visions of doom, and self-annihilating judgments—all of which can seem devastatingly real. "I cannot find a place for myself out there." "I've worked hard but my skills are useless." "There will never be anyone or anything for me." "I have nothing to offer anyone." "I'm boring, uninteresting, a drag. I am nothing."

This is no way to run a life, to be completely out of sync with reality! There is a place for everyone, though it does require you to participate in creating it. There are schools and classes. You can always increase your skills. People enter our lives from all directions in unpredictable ways, a fact that happily suggests the possibility of new personal connections.

The challenge is, how do you begin to alter your vision?

You do so in small manageable steps that do not require you to simply slice away old patterns of obsessively negative thought. That will never work. It's like starving yourself for five days and losing five pounds. You'll gain it right back. You should work toward altering your vision a bit at a time. And you have to start by recognizing the destructive patterns of thought that leave you entangled in an endless web of depressing perceptions.

BEWARE OF OVERGENERALIZING. When you're depressed, one mistake during a dinner conversation may leave you feeling like the bane of the dinner table. You might completely forget the smile you brought to someone's face a moment ago, or the possibility that you could do so again.

DON'T BE TOO RESPONSIBLE. You likely view yourself often as being the culprit behind the silence in a group, the bore in the business presentation, or the instigator of a fight with an intimate other. When you feel this way, ask yourself to slow down and think of where everyone else around you was. What were they doing? How did they participate? This is not to shift the blame. This is to share it.

REALIZE YOU'RE NOT CENTER STAGE. Depression can lead you to be so focused on yourself and your own shortcomings that it's easy to conclude that others too are completely focused on you and your imagined weaknesses. You might feel that every wart is magnified and everyone is struck by your ineptitude. But the truth is, when you're depressed and sticking to yourself, no one is noticing much of anything—not to mention one other critical thing . . .

REMEMBER, EVERYONE AROUND YOU HAS AN INTERNAL LIFE YOU DON'T KNOW ABOUT. This is extremely important to keep in mind. Depressed people tend to look out at the world and think, "Everyone's fine but me." But everyone isn't. It's not necessary to identify who is suffering silently along with you. But it is quite helpful to realize that you are not alone in the negative internal dialogue that is dragging you down.

There are many techniques for controlling (and eventually stopping) the obsessive thoughts that fuel your depression. These tools allow for the thoughts in a controlled fashion, leaving you free to analyze and even smile ruefully at them. Here are some suggestions:

DON'T MAKE A CATASTROPHE OUT OF EVERYTHING. If you say something that falls flat, or if a joke doesn't go over the way you expect it to, let it go. Don't dwell on it. Move on to the next topic of discussion.

DON'T MAKE IT ALL OR NOTHING. Don't expect perfection. Be proud of yourself for any progress you make along the way, and don't beat yourself up for any mishaps. Try to focus on the positive aspects of an experience.

DON'T THINK THAT YOU HAVE A SCARLET "D" ON YOUR CHEST. People who are depressed tend to think that everyone knows about their depression, but most people don't recognize the signs of depression in others. People have a way of hiding their problems, especially in social situations. Don't worry that you will be "found out." In all likelihood, given the high incidence of depression, you have friends and relatives who are also depressed, but you don't even know about it.

DON'T TURN ANGER INWARD. Depression can come from anger turned against the self. When you relentlessly blame and criticize yourself, you can become depressed. Self-criticism is an attack on the self, so we must ask, "Why on earth do we do that to ourselves?"

1. We learned to do it from being blamed or criticized excessively by others.
2. When we are hurt, we get quite angry. If the person who does the hurting is bigger or stronger or has control over us, it is dangerous to direct our anger toward him or her. So what do we do with our anger?
3. We divert anger away from the aggressor and turn it against ourselves in the form of self-criticism and self-blame.

How can you stop turning anger against yourself? Remember where the anger began; keep it connected to the original aggressor. Follow the anger; keep an edge on it to prevent it from turning against you.

SET ASIDE TIME TO ANALYZE DEPRESSING THOUGHTS. You cannot expect to just stop producing depressing thoughts. They are the creations of your worst fears and they need an outlet. To push them away guarantees their reappearance in some other negative form, like a violent temper or an even deeper depression than you already have. But you don't want them dogging your every step either. So schedule them. Pick a specific time frame—such as ten or twenty minutes—and give yourself a chance to wallow in your worst worries, fears, and anxieties. Indulge yourself, and when the allotted time is over, say to yourself, "I will get to you again either later today or tomorrow." Then, throughout the "off time" when these thoughts come up at you, gently remind yourself, "I'll see you later." This way you are not shutting yourself up. You're just adding some discipline to the picture. It's a good first step.

TAKE IT TO THE EXTREME AND BACK. Wrap yourself around the worry and analyze it to its most ridiculous level of panic, and then slowly bring it back again. Here's a shortened version: "I'm afraid I'll lose my job. Then what will happen? I'll end up on the street. Then what will you do? I'll have to find shelter, food. What will you do with the belongings in your house? I guess I'll have to give them all away. And what about your skills? What will you do with those? I guess I could find another job. How? I'll keep a few of my nice clothes for interviews . . ."

PUT IT IN WRITING. Creating inventories that examine your worst feelings can help. First you state the powerful fear and then the probable reality.

Next you admit to your weakness, and then note your strength. Finally you set out a reasonable expectation. Doing this will help you address the areas where you do need to work on yourself (pouring energy into denying a weakness will only make things worse), and keep what's positive about you in the light, where it inspires you to move forward and improve your self-esteem.

The depressing concern: I am a bore at parties. I can't talk.

The reality: Usually a few people end up chatting with me, though they don't look really interested.

My weakness: I am continually aware I'm not as scintillating in groups as other people I know. I feel inadequate. I keep wishing I were someone else.

My strength: I seem to be a pretty good listener. Even if I'm not talking and am just asking a question or two, people seem to want to tell me things. I like that. It takes the pressure off.

Goal: When someone is talking to me, I'd like to at least once or twice bring up something about me and then tell them about it, instead of just listening.

And finally, there's the Shock Yourself into Submission Technique, otherwise known as,

THE THOUGHT-STOPPING METHOD. Some people find this effective. When you notice you're having depressing thoughts, shout (either aloud or to yourself), *"No! Stop! Don't go there!"* Then, immediately focus your thoughts and attention on something more positive. Don't leave a blank space in your mind where depressing thoughts, like the seeds of weeds, can take root and flourish. At first you will find yourself shouting, *"No!"* many times, but eventually your *"No!"*'s will become stronger and less frequent.

Depressed people do tend to look at the world through dark gray glasses. You must learn to separate out what's truly troubling from what doesn't have to be, and that's what these tools help with. They allow you to keep the negative feelings from coloring everything.

The techniques you've just learned will be helpful, but another way to allow different perspectives into your life is to connect and communicate with others.

Step Out: Get Connected

Loneliness, feeling untethered to anyone or anything and yet aching for a closeness with someone, often permeates the existence of a depressed person. Unfortunately and ironically, most depressed people, in response to this agony, do exactly what they shouldn't. They curl up in a ball. Instead of moving outward they

do anything but reach out, and present such a per-
plexing and uninviting picture to those around them
that often they are deliberately left alone.

Most people enjoy it when they can successfully
comfort a friend, but too often depressed people are
unreachable. Either they stay resolutely engulfed in
their own hopeless vision of the world and thus shun
encouraging words, or they begin to turn off people
around them by accusing them of not understanding
their grief and struggles.

Ultimately they create the isolation that drives
them to despair, but are unable to see their own role in
their social undoing.

A pattern of isolation cannot be broken in a single
move. But there are things you can do to move out
into the world, opening up the possibility of a connection that can grow closer as time goes on.

JOIN A SUPPORT GROUP. Support groups, usually
run by a clinician who specializes in issues of depression, include other depression sufferers who are
well aware of the way you are feeling. They know
better than to expect more from you than you can
handle. You will likely hear their stories, and not
only will you be comforted by the commonalities
between you, but the isolation you feel will melt
away.

JOIN A RELIGIOUS GROUP. Research has shown
that people who gather together around common

beliefs and spiritual activities are much less prone to depression. Human beings naturally have an urge to reach outside of their daily lives to connect with something greater than themselves. As an added benefit, joining this kind of organization brings you into contact with people on a level that feels not invasive but mutually enriching.

NURTURE SOMEONE OR SOMETHING ELSE. The ability to nurture, protect, and sustain someone or something else can help to create a sense of self-worth. Feeling needed is tremendously rewarding, but depressed people often feel woefully expendable. Caring for a pet, volunteering to help in a soup kitchen, or helping out in a nursing home not only is very much appreciated by those on the receiving end but allows the caregiver to feel fulfilled and nurtured as well. In military writings, one sees that prisoners of war increase their chances of survival if they have a pet . . . whether it is a rat or even a few flies. Sustaining someone or something else requires that you take a piece of yourself and offer it up. It is a small but significant release from the self-centered aspect of your depression.

There are other ways of combating this isolation that can give you healthy outlets for the many positive and negative emotions within you.

MAKE SOMETHING:
EXPRESSIVE OUTLETS

Depression uses a lot of juice. Once it has gone through your most negative thoughts, it begins plundering your deeper ones. When those get disrupted, your positive self can easily be engulfed by the misery. Eventually, the part of you from which so many ideas spring, and in which new choices are made, satisfying solutions are found, and art of any form is appreciated and conceived, will begin to founder.

This "part" is your inner or creative self, and you must protect it. *It is yours and yours alone.* It is an essential determinant of who you are, how you experience and generate pleasure, and how you grow intellectually and emotionally. Perhaps most important, in terms of depression, it is a powerful weapon. Our creative self builds. Our depression rips things apart. As much as possible, you need to bring your imaginative and resourceful self to bear on your destructive inclinations.

Too often, in our modern society, we focus on strengthening the outer self and ignore the inner self. We become fixated on success, money, and taking care of our families, but this doesn't bring us peace of mind. While the outer self thrives, the inner self withers. A fulfilling life is about achieving balance. Although it's important to meet your responsibilities to others, you must also take care of yourself. Tapping into your creative inner self can help you flourish in ways you never thought possible.

At this point you might be thinking, "Well, I'm not an inventor, an artist, or a musician. I can't design and build a new bridge, and I don't write." But self-expression and creativity can be given voice through any activity that brings you peace or transports you to a place where the task at hand is all that matters.

I'm speaking of cooking, gardening, flower arranging, language classes, bird-watching, fishing, any form of collecting.

When you immerse yourself in an interest, a few things are happening. You take a vacation from the sense of worthlessness you experience. You nurture that part of yourself that can still feel healthfully involved, and you do something totally for you. An artistic activity may allow you to vent a hurt feeling, but you will do so in a positive way. There need be no intent to please anyone but yourself, though of course it's nice if you do bring pleasure to others. Time will pass quickly. When you step away from the endeavor, you will likely feel refreshed for having immersed yourself in building rather than tearing apart.

Giving yourself over to an interest or expressing yourself through an artistic or intellectual endeavor will feel as if you have let something clear, good, and without boundary into your life. Internally you will step out of the box of depression. You will let your mind travel to another place.

It's time to look at how your physical self can do the same.

Body Depression

Your body, especially when it comes to depression, has an astounding ability to reflect how you feel emotionally. The way it does this is different for everyone, depending on the way you are physiologically wired. Everyone's brain chemistry has its own unique profile. The fact remains that the mind and body exert tremendous influence over each other. Though we may not know absolutely in what order this occurs at any moment in time, we do know that together they play a key role in the maelstrom of depression.

Quite simply, the body houses an enormous stockpile of physical and emotional stress. You must relieve your physical self of this tension in order to gain control over your emotions.

EXERCISE

There is good evidence that exercise can improve mood, though exactly how it does so remains unclear. Of the two possible explanations, one is psychological and the other physiological.

Psychologically speaking, exercise can be a powerful diversion. You have to step away from work and other stresses to engage in a sport of any kind, and in so doing, you temporarily remove yourself from the onslaught of worry and pressure.

Physiologically, it is believed that anxiety and depression are the results of complex electrical and bio-chemical processes in the brain. Exercise has a positive effect on mood by increasing blood flow to the brain, stimulating the nervous system through electrical impulses, and raising levels of every mood-related neurotransmitter, including endorphins—our brain's own painkillers.

I believe that the boost from exercise is the direct result of both psychological and physiological factors. The symbolic meaning of the activity, the distraction from worries, the acquisition of mastery, the effect on self-image, and the chemical changes all play parts.

Frequent exercise is also an effective treatment for anxiety and, according to some research, can be as effective as psychotherapy in treating mild depression. Although aerobic exercise offers the greatest cardiovascular benefit, any form of enjoyable exercise can give you a psychological lift and help counteract the impact of stress in your life.

A word of caution, however, concerning the competitive spirit. It's alive in most of us, but it doesn't necessarily make us well. If you are seeking to use exercise to relieve tension, then it might be wise to select an activity where you don't have to win or lose, or even feel responsible for someone else's win or loss (doubles tennis, for example). The idea is that the exercise be its own end, and not just the pursuit of a winning score.

At this point you might be worrying, "I don't have

the energy to take up a new sport or to throw myself into spiffy exercise togs and climb onto all the equipment at the local gym that looks more like medieval torture devices than anything else."

So take a walk. You don't need special clothes or equipment. The perceived exertion is low, but the actual benefit is high. In other words, you don't have to work at it, but it will work for you. People tend not to drop out of walking. It can be done anytime, anywhere, and it can reduce the level of stress in the body considerably. Walking outside instead of on an indoor track makes it easier to focus outward. And you gain an additional bonus because fresh air and sunlight have beneficial effects on depression.

Your body and mind are inextricably linked. Exercise will undoubtedly help you gain some control over your depression. Physically your tension will recede, while physiologically the levels of brain chemicals which help relieve anxiety and improve mood will increase. And then too there's the simple fact that making the decision to put on a pair of sneakers, go outside, and exert yourself is a way of reminding yourself that you deserve to feel better and that you can take charge of your recovery.

Relaxation Techniques

Depression is typically characterized by a seemingly dull thought pattern, laggard movements, an absence of energy, and a profound turn inward, but the truth is that it is a state of high excitation. Sufferers may feel hopeless, stuck, caught in quicksand, and beaten, but they are anything but calm. In fact, they are in a panic. Though exercise can relieve tension in the body, relaxation techniques such as breathing exercises, meditation, and Yoga have a profound effect on bringing the body and mind into connectedness and a more relaxed state.

Herbert Benson published *The Relaxation Response* in 1975 as a study of the effect of transcendental meditation on the body. This book has become one of the most important works available for people dealing with stress, anxiety, and depression. By concentrating on the disciplines of exercise, breathing, and posture, Benson discovered that regular meditation, which he referred to as "deep relaxation," led to a number of positive physical changes. In the short run there was a decrease in heart rate, respiration, blood pressure, and muscle tension, accompanied by an increase in alpha wave activity in the brain. Over the long run, he found, regular deep relaxation resulted in a reduction of anxiety, an increase in feelings of well-being, and important cardiovascular improvements.

THE RELAXATION RESPONSE

There are a number of ways to achieve what has become known as the Relaxation Response, and they are easy to teach yourself. Here is a thumbnail sketch that should get you started:

1. Find a quiet spot with a comfortable place to sit or lie down.
2. Sit upright either on a pad in a Yoga position (legs crossed) or in a comfortable chair with your feet on the floor and your back supported. Close your eyes.
3. Spend a few minutes focusing on the points of muscle tension in your body, willing the tension away and imagining it replaced by warmth.
4. Concentrate on your breaths, counting them and making them as regular as possible. You might then choose to focus on a word or phrase that has meaning for you.
5. Adopt a passive attitude. Visualize a tranquil pool. When thoughts intrude into your consciousness, visualize them as bubbles in the pool rising to the surface and gently dissipating.
6. Avoid self-consciousness. Do not evaluate how you are doing. Simply concentrate on your rhythmic breathing.
7. Do this for about ten to twenty minutes. When you finish, sit quietly for a minute or so with your eyes closed. Do not stand for one or two minutes.

PROGRESSIVE MUSCLE RELAXATION

There are other ways of achieving relaxation, including progressive muscle relaxation, in which you move methodically through your body, tensing and then relaxing each major muscle group. This helps you to become more sensitized to the different feelings specific muscles radiate as they tense or relax. It can be done in a large chair but is best done while lying on your back on a firm but soft surface.

1. Loosen your clothing and lie with your arms along your sides.
2. First tense the muscles throughout your body from head to toe. Tighten your feet and legs, tense your arms and hands, clench your jaw, and contract your stomach. Hold these and other muscles tightly while you feel the strain. Then take a deep breath, hold it, and exhale slowly as you relax all your muscles, letting go of the tension.
3. You can then do the same for individual groups of muscles. Start by making your hands into tight fists. Feel the tension, relax, and let go. Do the same with your arms, pressing them down against the surface you're resting on. Feel the tension. Hold it and let go, continuing on to the next group of muscles.
4. Finally, experience your whole body at rest, letting go of all tension. Allow yourself to enjoy this state

of relaxation and peace for a few minutes before standing up.

Mindfulness Meditation

Usually the notion of meditation conjures up words like "mantra" and the idea that any thought that comes up at you is a distraction to be brushed away.

Mindfulness meditation, also known as insight meditation, is another major classification of meditation practice. The ultimate goal of this kind of meditation is acceptance, which does not mean giving in to difficulties but rather moving along with them—rolling with the punches, if you will. Mindfulness meditation helps you to observe what is going on in your mind and remove all judgments as you are aware of the thoughts and feelings that come in and out of your consciousness. By noting all of the thoughts that cross your mind without allowing yourself to get stuck with heavy emotion on any of them, you will gain a new perspective on everything that is happening in your life, both good and bad.

You begin by concentrating on any one thought to achieve a sense of calmness and centeredness. Once this is achieved, you can begin to broaden your range of observation. When thoughts or feelings come up in your mind, do not ignore them, push them away, analyze them, or judge them. Rather, simply note the thoughts as they occur, focusing attention on how different thoughts move in and out of each other. In so doing, you may become less caught up with these thoughts and gain a deeper understanding of your reactions to everyday stress and pressures. Mindfulness is essentially a simple moment-to-moment awareness and can be practiced while showering, chatting, eating, painting, or shaving!

The nonjudgmental aspect of this meditation is critical. In the absence of editing and censoring, you can more clearly see the content of your thoughts and identify the feelings associated with them. This quiet, accepting observance can help you gain insight into what is behind much of your depression. In short, it helps you to stand apart from negative patterns of thought and begin moving out of the dark tunnel in which you have been laboring.

There is an excellent book that I recommend to my patients who are interested in learning more about meditation: *Living From the Heart: Heart Rhythm Meditation for Energy, Clarity, Peace, Joy and Inner Power* by Puran Bair (Three Rivers Press, New York, 1998). This book details a very simple method for learning meditation, and is particularly good for novices.

Yoga

Yoga is a complete science of life that originated in India many thousands of years ago. It is the oldest system of personal healthful development in the world and embraces the body, mind, and spirit. Here I seek only to present an overall picture of how the practice of Yoga might help you to reach for a depression-free life. There are many books devoted entirely to this broad and complex discipline and all kinds of classes available to lead you through the techniques. If you wish to discover Yoga, I urge you to explore the many resources available.

The Yoga postures *(asanas)* exercise and stimulate every part of the body, stretching and toning muscles, joints, spine, and skeletal system. They also work on the internal organs, glands, and nerves, keeping these systems healthy. By relieving physical and consequently mental tension, the *asanas* also release vast resources of energy.

The Yoga breathing exercises, known as *pranayama,* revitalize the body and help to control the mind. You are left feeling calm and refreshed. The meditation aspect of Yoga results in increased clarity, mental power, and ability to concentrate.

Recently medical research has begun to focus more attention on Yoga. Studies have shown that relaxation in the Corpse Pose (lying on your back with your arms and legs stretched out) lowers high blood pressure, and that regular practice of *asanas* and *pranayama* can improve arthritis, arteriosclerosis, chronic fatigue, and heart conditions. Laboratory tests have also confirmed Yoga's influence over autonomic, or involuntary, functions such as heart rate and blood pressure.

There are three essential parts to relaxation through the practice of Yoga: physical, mental, and spiritual. For a taste of this, assume the Corpse Pose, tensing and then relaxing each part of the body in turn (just as I described under Relaxation Response techniques). It is believed that this tensing and relaxing is essential for you to be sure you have indeed achieved the full relaxation you are capable of. With practice, you will be able to use your mind to send messages to your involuntary muscles, such as the heart and digestive system. To relax the mind, breathe steadily and rhythmically, making use of all parts of your lungs to increase your intake of oxygen. The spiritual relaxation comes when you can detach yourself, becoming a witness to your own body and mind. Obviously these higher states of relaxation will take some time to achieve. Again, I urge you to seek out a Yoga class or reference.

The practice of Yoga includes a proper diet of well-balanced natural food to keep the body light and supple and the mind calm. Positive thinking and meditation help to remove negative thoughts and still the mind. The Yoga technique of relaxation will give you feelings of expansion, lightness, and a warm glow. When all muscular tension is gone, you will be filled with a sense of well-being. Relaxation in Yoga is not a particular state as much as it is a process composed of an ever-increasing depth of peaceful wholeness. It centers on the idea of letting go, instead of holding on. As you relax your whole body and breathe slowly, physiological changes occur, including the release of muscle tension, a decrease in activity of the sympathetic nervous system, and an increase in parasympathetic activity. Just a few minutes of deep relaxation will reduce worry and fatigue.

The *asanas,* which form the foundation of a daily practice of Yoga, are said to reawaken your awareness and control of your body, and they have the spiritual effect of freeing you from fears so that you may find confidence and serenity.

Proper breathing, another aspect of Yoga, may regulate the brain stem and the vagal nerve input to the brain. But proper breathing is not limited to Yoga alone. This kind of breathing changes the acid-base balance in the body and alters the way anxiety-regulating nerves function. There is a worry center in the brain stem called the Locus Ceruleus, and here breathing exerts a calming influence.

Most people have forgotten how to breathe properly. They breathe shallowly through the mouth and make little or no use of the diaphragm, either lifting the shoulders or contracting the abdomen when they inhale. In this way only a small amount of oxygen can be taken in and only the top of the lungs is used, resulting, it is believed, in a lack of vitality and low resistance to disease. When you are angry or scared your breathing is shallow, rapid, and irregular. Conversely, when you are relaxed or deep in thought your breathing becomes rich and slow.

The practice of Yoga demands that you reverse poor breathing habits. Breathing correctly means breathing through the nose, keeping the mouth closed, and performing a full inhalation and exhalation, bringing the whole of your lungs into play. There are many different kinds of Yoga breathing exercises, including forced exhalation, which rids the lower lungs of stale air, and alternate-nostril breathing, in which you inhale through one nostril at a time. Both of these exercises are meant to bring your life force (energy) into balance.

Therapeutic Help

This chapter has been about what you can do to take control of your depression. Not all of these techniques work for everyone. You may need to try several to see which work best for you. Hopefully, you will be able to use the techniques described here to at least manage the degree of your depression, so that you can begin to heal. For some of you, the depression-proofing techniques described, combined with the other three dimensions, will keep you depression-free. Others, however, may need or want more help.

If you feel that you do not want to do this portion of the Stop Depression Now program alone, you can seek help from a cognitive behavioral therapist, a psychologist, or a physician who specializes in treating depression by changing people's thought patterns. These are therapists who are skilled in helping people utilize the techniques we have described in this chapter. For a referral to a cognitive behavioral therapist, call the Beck Institute of Cognitive Therapy at (610) 664-3020 or the American Institute of Cognitive Therapy at (212) 308-2440.

People are susceptible to depression for a variety of reasons, and some of these causes do not have their origin in brain chemistry. Some are born of early childhood traumas, inadequate grieving, and even feelings of anger and frustration over circumstances which we cannot allow ourselves to know are unbearably painful. Many "identified" causes of depression ("I hate my work," "My lover left me") are often symbols for the real, more deep-rooted cause, and this is where so-called "talking cures" come in. Therapeutic intervention—that is, seeking help from a psychiatrist or psychologist—can help you to uncover the actual source of pain that is behind the depression. I bring this up here because, in a way, seeking therapy of some kind is a way of taking control. It requires your participation and commitment, but it can be tremendously fruitful in stopping a never-ending pattern of depressive episodes.

The bottom line is that there is no one road you can take toward being depression-free—no magic wand. You have to bring your whole self to the task. If you begin by taking baby steps and accept the need for small lifestyle changes, after a while, change will become easier, and what feel like tiny steps will be great leaps forward.

Part 3

SAM-e for Special Situations

9

Good News for Women: New Hope for Postpartum and Menopausal Depression

Approximately twenty-five percent of women—compared to twelve percent of men—suffer from clinical depression, beginning most often in adolescence. Depression is the single most common emotional disorder in women. About one fourth of women have a major bout of depression at some time in their lives. Why is the rate of depression so much higher in women than in men?

It may simply be due to the fact that women are more likely to express their feelings than men are. Physically designed to be child-bearers and socially positioned as child-rearers, women are more naturally attuned to feelings, to the nuances of emotions and biological needs. This is not to say that these qualities are bad: the survival of the species probably depended on them! If a mother did not respond to the needs of an infant—if she did not recognize the cues of hunger or distress—there would be little chance of that child surviving long-term. This was especially true back in our hunter-gatherer days, when women were often the sole caretakers of children. Without caring mothers, the human species would not have gotten very far.

Modern women may have an expanded role in society beyond motherhood, but because of it, they are often likely to be torn in different directions. Many are now both breadwinners and bread makers, putting in long days that can be stressful and exhausting. The lot of the homemaker is often no better, since she is the one who takes care of everyone else at home, runs the local school board, but doesn't have the time (or often the resources) to meet her own needs. The chronic stress of having to be there for everybody can exact a steep toll on the psyche. Because women can speak comfortably about emotional issues, they are more likely to ask for help in coping with their problems.

This doesn't mean that real men don't get depressed. Not at all! Men often deal with depression differently, either masking it or submerging it in work and competition or, more destructively, in substance abuse, gambling, and high-risk behaviors.

Biological danger zones and environmental triggers also play complex and powerful roles in the high rate of depression in women between the ages of thirty-five and sixty-five. The American Medical Women's Association has identified the periods of a woman's life when her likelihood of becoming depressed increases. It's not surprising to learn that those times coincide with increased hormonal activity and with extraordinary life changes that challenge even the finest coping skills.

Depression seems to occur more frequently after childbirth, and before, during, and after menopause. This is due to hormonal factors and to the stress—both positive and negative—that accompanies any major life change.

But there's more good news about SAM-e that can help women arrive at, work through, and emerge from these turning points less depressed and more at ease with their lives.

Postpartum Depression

About fifty to eighty percent of all new mothers experience some postpartum blues. This number is so high as to suggest that some symptoms of depression, such as mood swings and crying, are normal following the intensity of childbirth. They usually go away within a week or two.

But an estimated ten to fifteen percent of new mothers have more significant and persistent problems that don't disappear so quickly. Many of the symptoms of postpartum depression are very similar to those of depression, among them loss of appetite, inability to sleep despite being exhausted, irritability, sadness, and anxiety, and they can deprive your first few months of motherhood of the joys you expected.

Postpartum depression leads some women to feel inadequate as mothers, fearful for their children, and unable to maintain their other relationships. In severe cases it can lead to obsessive-compulsive disorder, in which a mother cannot let go of thoughts of harm coming to her child, sometimes even from herself—thoughts which shock and depress her still more.

During and after pregnancy, a woman must integrate the new role of motherhood into her identity. This raises a whole series of personal issues: "Who am I? What is my concept of motherhood? How do I feel about my new role?" The concept of the ideal mother you would like to be must be balanced with the person you know you are. The expectations of spouses and family members can have particular significance during this time of life. Having help and support from family members in the first few months of your baby's life may be helpful, but their increased presence may also raise other emotional issues. It can be a time of confusion. And the expectation that this should be a time of bliss can add further pressure to an already fragile state.

If there is a history of depression in your family or you've suffered from depression yourself in your life, you are more likely to face postpartum depression. If you were depressed following one birth, you're more likely to suffer again with subsequent births.

The most significant contributor to all depression

and therefore to postpartum depression is stress. Whether the stress is positive—the sheer excitement of a new life in your home—or negative—a lack of financial or emotional support—the stress itself is enough to make you depressed. The process of bringing a new person into a household is such a big change that, as one study noted, even adoptive parents can be prone to depression. And the emotional high of expecting the child turns into the daunting reality of parenthood for all new parents. Depression can result.

There is evidence that miscarriage can lead to postpartum depression. This is something women should discuss with their doctors.

One aspect of teenage pregnancy that has received little attention despite all the discussion of the problem is that about thirty-five percent of teen mothers suffer from postpartum depression. Another study indicates that more than ten percent of fathers suffer from some form of depression in the postnatal period. So even though we tend to focus on problems of new mothers, the emotional needs of new fathers should not be neglected, especially those who are depression-prone.

GET HELP

In the past, many women suffered in silence with postpartum depression, feeling ashamed and inadequate, embarrassed to admit they were having problems with motherhood. Fortunately, those days are over.

Still, you may feel that your difficulties will end soon and that you haven't got the time or the energy to take care of yourself when you have a newborn to care for. This delay in dealing with postpartum depression won't make it go away.

Just having someone to talk to always helps. And beyond that, your doctor may be able to refer you to a therapist if you don't already have one. Psychotherapists can evaluate whether an antidepressant is in order.

SAM-E OFFERS HOPE

SAM-e can be an effective tool in dealing with postpartum depression, with one important caveat. Studies have shown that more than half of all women who suffer from serious postpartum depression are prone to bipolar depression. Therefore an antidepressant may aggravate this condition. Before taking SAM-e or any other antidepressant, women with postpartum depression should be evaluated by a physician.

For many women, SAM-e may prove to be the right treatment. Initial studies have shown it to be effective in reducing or relieving the signs and symptoms of postpartum depression. In a study conducted in 1993, two groups of thirty patients each were compared. One group of new mothers were given 1600mg a day of SAM-e, while the others were given a placebo. After thirty days of treatment, the patients receiving SAM-e showed a significant improvement in mood and a reduction in both depression and anxiety.

The gynecologic and obstetric department of the University of Padua in Italy also conducted a study of sixty women whose age, type of delivery, and marital status were similar. Two days after delivery the patients completed a symptom questionnaire. Those with scores indicating psychological distress were selected and assigned to a double-blind treatment with either SAM-e or a placebo. Two 400mg tablets of SAM-e were taken daily by one group, while the other took placebos. The patients were evaluated ten days and thirty days after delivery, using the symptom questionnaire.

By the tenth day, the group taking SAM-e felt far fewer symptoms of depression than those on the placebo. By the thirtieth day, the results were dramatic, leading the researchers at the University of Padua to conclude that SAM-e is a valuable and effective treatment for reducing or relieving the symptoms of postpartum depression. Moreover, this relief occurred in a relatively short period of time.

With the arrival of SAM-e in the United States, women can find significant help for postpartum depression. Most patients taking SAM-e report a dramatic increase in energy levels, a report I hear more often for SAM-e than for any other antidepressant. New mothers can certainly use more energy. Because SAM-e acts quickly, women can find relief when they need it most: as soon as the postpartum depression strikes. And since SAM-e has no notable side effects, women can feel comfortable choosing it and increasing the dosage when necessary until the depression departs.

IF YOU ARE BREAST-FEEDING

Whatever nutrients and substances you take into your body find their way into your breast milk and therefore into your baby. Everything you eat or ingest must therefore be examined as to its effect on your baby, not just now but years from now as well.

As we have seen, SAM-e is a naturally occurring substance within the human body, and babies have a high level of it in their systems. Also, high doses of SAM-e have been used to treat pregnant women with gallstones without causing any apparent problems to their babies. This would suggest that SAM-e is safe for breast-feeding mothers. Again, a word of caution however: SAM-e has not been extensively studied in breast-feeding women. In fact, there is only limited data about antidepressants in general in breast-feeding women.

Some women who suffer from depression during pregnancy have been able to obtain significant relief from prescription antidepressants. Studies have been conducted, for example, which conclude that Prozac is safe during pregnancy, but not enough research has been done on its safety during breast-feeding. For instance, high levels of Prozac are passed through breast milk. We believe that Zoloft is safe during breast-feeding because very little is passed through to the breast milk.

On the other hand, these other antidepressants can take a long time to work, and they have significant side effects. SAM-e may be the best choice for the breast-feeding mother who needs help with postpartum depression, because of its quick action and lack of side effects. However, I urge you to make your decision in consultation with your doctor. More studies will answer the question as SAM-e becomes better-known in the United States.

As an aside, you may recall how important DHA is in our depression-fighting diet. But do not overlook its role in helping your baby grow strong—and smart! Consider boosting your DHA intake while you are breast-feeding. This will give your little one the best start possible.

Menopause and Depression

Menopause is a time of enormous hormonal change in the female body. Beginning with the erratic and inconsistent periods that characterize perimenopause and continuing through to the end of menstruation altogether, menopause represents the biggest change in a woman's body and life since her first menstrual period.

Hormonal changes are enough to cause some depression. Estrogen is decreased dramatically during menopause. Because estrogen is known to modulate serotonin and dopamine, menopausal women are going to be more prone to the kind of depression caused by hormonal changes.

If a woman has a vulnerability to depression or has been depressed in the past, she is at a slightly higher risk during peri- or postmenopause.

There is some controversy, however, about regarding menopausal women as necessarily prone to depression or assuming that menopause itself is a cause of depression.

Although many women do experience mood changes around the time of menopause, a link with clinical depression has not been determined. Sleep disturbances, anxiety, some irritability, and other symptoms arise that look like depression, but these can just as easily be attributable to other factors in a woman's life at midlife. The forties and fifties are a time of reevaluation. There are bound to be some regrets and losses that reveal themselves more fully when you are contemplating where you've been and where you might be going. Midlife is also a time when children have left home (or may return home as adults). Marriages may end or go through serious changes. Careers can shift either through downsizing or from your own desire to branch out and try new things. Elderly parents may require more care and attention. Family and friends may be ill or passing on. You're about to face the fact that you're aging and not immortal. All of these milestones are challenging and unsettling. It's easy to see why some people associate this time with depression.

Our culture of youth disregards older women. That is changing as millions of baby-boomer women enter menopause. This generation will redefine old age in the same way it has redefined every other stage of life in America in the past half century.

So don't assume that menopause is going to make you depressed. But if you find that you *are* depressed or if you want to help yourself make this life transition a more positive experience, read on.

SAM-E AND MENOPAUSE— A PROMISING PARTNERSHIP

If depression does strike during menopause, it will not differ in any significant way from ordinary depression. That's good news, because SAM-e can help at this time of life in all the ways it helps anyone suffering from depression. What's more, SAM-e can help with menopause even if you aren't depressed.

The controversy about hormone replacement therapy (HRT) is still ongoing. Many women are left uncertain about whether they wish to take HRT at all. You can certainly use SAM-e safely with this therapy. If you decide against it, or while you're considering the decision, SAM-e can offer at least one of the benefits of estrogen replacement: SAM-e acts quickly to regulate mood swings—faster, in fact, than prescription antidepressants, and with minimal or no side effects.

Many women find that SAM-e greatly reduces menopausally related sleep disturbances. Everything in life is easier to deal with when you've had the restorative night's sleep that SAM-e helps to provide. Moreover, night sweats may be less likely to awaken you as often when you're in a deep sleep.

SAM-e's numerous antiaging properties shine at a time when slowing down the aging process is particularly important. SAM-e can potentially lower the risk of heart attack and stroke, which rises dramatically after menopause. It appears to protect the joints from osteoarthritis, as we discuss in Chapter 11 ("Getting Healthy with SAM-e"). It may protect the nerves from deterioration, which will help maintain mental acuity, and seems to help the aging brain (also see Chapter 11).

Taking care of the body in this positive way makes you an active participant in the care of your own life and longevity. During menopause, it is more important than ever to exercise, to practice healthful nutrition, and to avail yourself of stress-reduction techniques. Don't neglect Steps 3 and 4 of the Stop Depression Now program! With increased energy and less depression, you'll be more motivated to take good care of yourself. It's never too late to incorporate positive changes in lifestyle. Even if in the past you've been less than vigilant in taking care of yourself, start now. The results will be rewarding.

10

At Last! Relief for Fibromyalgia

"The good news is it doesn't kill you . . . and the bad news is it doesn't kill you."

PATIENT WITH FIBROMYALGIA

Up to 10 million Americans suffer from fibromyalgia, a syndrome that has been around for most of the century but is just now beginning to get recognition and attention in the medical community. A chronic pain disorder, fibromyalgia is characterized by widespread muscle aches, stiffness, and general fatigue and is often accompanied by depression. The term itself means pain in the fibrous tissue, but the exact cause is still unknown.

Women—often in their early-to-mid-thirties— account for ninety percent of fibromyalgia cases. The median age of diagnosis extends into the fifties, meaning that many patients suffer for years before receiving an accurate diagnosis.

Until now, there have been few options for fibromyalgia sufferers. The medicines prescribed for it range from sedatives to stimulants, from ordinary ibuprofen to prescription beta-blockers and hormones. Each of these has side effects and not all have been effective. Encouragingly, in an area very much in need of encouraging news, SAM-e can help relieve the pain and depression of fibromyalgia for many. There are several scientific studies that attest to its effectiveness, as well as our own clinical experience with patients.

There is no cure for fibromyalgia. Until recently, there was little agreement in the medical community that the problem even existed. To patients as well as doctors, fibromyalgia can be as frustrating as it is confounding. As noted above, it can take years to get a definitive diagnosis. In the past, when patients complained about how tired, sore, and defeated they felt, their doctors would be quick to dismiss these symptoms. After all, physicians were presented with patients who had persistent symptoms but no obvious physiological causes. Additionally, most of the sufferers were women in their thirties, forties, and fifties, while most of the medical establishment was made up of men generally much older than their patients. These older, male doctors were not accustomed to seeing female patients with jobs and careers, husbands and children, tight schedules and a myriad of responsibilities that women hadn't had before. Why shouldn't these women be sore, tired, and demoralized? The fact that they had been running at sixty miles per hour before, but now couldn't rev up to ten, didn't seem at all surprising. Many doctors either told them to slow down and feel okay about it—something that wasn't necessarily an option—or told them they were fine while privately regarding them as somewhat out of control and hysterical. In short, either "Live with it," or "It's all in your head."

As in depression, biochemical imbalances such as low serotonin levels also play a role in many cases of fibromyalgia. A decrease in serotonin leads to a shortage of refreshing sleep and an increase in pain sensitivity. Some doctors would recommend treatment for depression—not a bad idea, considering that depression appeared to be one component of the problem. But the problem was much more than depression.

Making matters even more complicated, the very symptoms these patients complained of would wax and wane. Patients would begin to feel better, and try to resume their normal activities. Within a week they'd be back in bed, feeling hopeless and guilty. As if the aches and pains, stiffness, swelling in soft tissue, tender points, and muscle spasms weren't enough, the pain was almost constant. Medications didn't help much with the neurological problems that accompanied the physical ones—the forgetfulness, sudden lack of coordination, and propensity to lose and drop things. In turn, these aspects would make people lose confidence in themselves and perhaps restrict social interactions, the very activities that make life fun.

Fibromyalgia symptoms would often change: A patient might have pain but lots of energy, saying she could deal with the soreness as long as she could maintain her life. Then the pain would become so great as to consume all her energy. Even the more specific symptoms a patient might complain of, like a sore throat or swelling of the lymph nodes, are conditions doctors see all the time. There was no consistency to the problem. It was difficult to diagnose and deal with effectively.

Fibromyalgia is not considered a disease in the conventional sense. Doctors cannot test for it in the usual ways—by taking X rays, drawing blood, or ordering a CAT scan or MRI. Yet people can undergo numerous time-consuming tests that show normal results, leading to even more frustration and despair. Moreover, many of the symptoms of fibromyalgia can be attributed to a wide range of conditions. Difficulty concentrating or performing simple mental tasks, and numbness or tingling suggest numerous other problems.

Getting to a Diagnosis

Fortunately, doctors can no longer ignore this increasingly common ailment. The pain in the muscles and the tendons and ligaments connecting them can now be identified and quantified by a test established in 1990 by the American College of Rheumatology. In what's known as a tender point exam, physicians evaluate how much pain occurs when pressure is applied to eighteen tender points near the neck, knees, elbows, and hips. If at least eleven of the eighteen points are sensitive, if the pain has lingered for at least three months, and if no other illness can be found, doctors can diagnose fibromyalgia.

Taking a good family medical history also helps identify the problem. Recent research suggests a genetic predisposition to chronic fatigue syndrome and fibromyalgia. A family history of chemical sensitivities, emotional problems, musculoskeletal problems, sleep pattern disturbances, and autoimmune diseases such as lupus can also alert a physician that fibromyalgia is a possibility.

Fibromyalgia is one of the components of chronic fatigue syndrome—an equally misunderstood problem that is as frustrating as it is widespread. Chronic fatigue syndrome is defined as persistent or relapsing fatigue neither attributable to ongoing exercise nor relieved by rest, and not due to other illnesses. Although chronic fatigue syndrome and fibromyalgia are talked about as two separate diseases, many patients have symptoms of both.

SAM-e Brings Hope and Help

Of all the symptoms of fibromyalgia, depression and soreness are the most stubborn to deal with. Now dramatic evidence has emerged that SAM-e can be effective in relieving the kind of depression and muscle soreness that specifically result from fibromyalgia. The addition of this natural supplement to the treatment of fibromyalgia is a major discovery—one that has been confirmed in numerous studies—that can make a real and lasting difference.

People with fibromyalgia may not be clinically depressed. More likely their depression comes from having the fibromyalgia in the first place. My experience has shown fibromyalgia patients to be angry at the disease itself. In the past, their only options were the chemical antidepressants like Prozac, Zoloft, and others. Because fibromyalgia sufferers are already taking various medications to ease their symptoms, adding these strong chemicals can have different side effects than cause in other people.

By being able to use SAM-e, a natural substance with no significant side effects, fibromyalgia patients get the best of all worlds—relief from depression and muscle soreness without side effects or possible adverse interactions with other medications.

Since SAM-e has been available in Europe for many years, that is where the research into its use for fibromyalgia has taken place. All of these studies proved it to be safe and effective in relieving the depression and soreness associated with fibromyalgia.

• In 1987, in a double-blind crossover study involving seventeen patients at the Institute of Medical Pathology I, Rheumatic Disease Unit, University of Pisa, Italy, doctors first reported that SAM-e could help reduce the symptoms of fibromyalgia. For twenty-one days, one group of patients were given 200mg of SAM-e per day while another group were given placebos. Two weeks later, following a "washout" period of no medicine, the groups were switched. The results were dramatic. In both cases, those patients taking SAM-e noticed a significant improvement in mood and outlook whereas those on the placebo did not obtain similar effects. The doctors concluded, "SAM-e treatment, by improving the depressive state and reducing the number of trigger points, seems to be an effective and safe therapy in the management of primary fibromyalgia." (*American Journal of Medicine,* November 20, 1987, Vol. 83, supp. 5A.)

• In 1991, doctors in the departments of rheumatology at hospitals in Copenhagen and Frederiksberg, Denmark, conducted a study involving forty-four patients with primary fibromyalgia. Half the group were given SAM-e (800mg a day orally) and the other half were given a placebo. After six weeks, patients taking SAM-e experienced reduced morning stiffness, decreased tenderness at their trigger points, and improvement in mood as compared to those taking the placebo. The researchers concluded, "S-adenosylmethionine [SAM-e] has some beneficial effects on primary fibromyalgia and could be an important option in the treatment." (*Scandinavian Journal of Rheumatology*, 1991: 20, 294–302.)

- In a later Italian study involving forty-seven patients with primary fibromyalgia, researchers gave patients SAM-e for six weeks. "The results of our clinical trial indicate that SAM-e effectively relieves the signs and symptoms of PF [primary fibromyalgia], while beneficially influencing the depressive mood associated with this condition . . . Although its mechanism of action is yet unknown, SAM-e has proved to be effective in relieving pain and impaired mood in patients with PF." An added, unexpected benefit: Patients reported that SAM-e improved the quality of their sleep, probably due to pain relief. (*Current Therapeutic Research*, July 1994, Vol. 55, No. 7.)

- Other studies done in Italy between 1994 and 1998 confirmed the emerging good news. Not only was SAM-e effective in improving the depressive mood and muscle soreness associated with fibromyalgia, its side effects were generally negligible.

Many of my patients who have been taking SAM-e for fibromyalgia report that it has helped them more than anything else. From 200 to 800mg a day of

SAM-e (and in rare cases, more), sometimes in combination with other prescriptions, sometimes alone, have had a big impact on the quality of their lives and on their ability to cope with the continued presence of fibromyalgia. I am very gratified to see these results, as I hope other doctors will be.

And because SAM-e usually has no negative side effects, doctors can increase dosage recommendations when necessary—something they cannot do as easily with other antidepressants or pain-relieving medications.

Fibromyalgia is a difficult syndrome which is only now becoming better understood. We don't know the cause and we don't have a cure. This makes the discovery of SAM-e as a treatment for the syndrome all the more important. For patients who went undiagnosed for years while desperately wondering what was wrong with themselves and for patients who now know they have a syndrome that may never go away, the proof of SAM-e's effectiveness in dealing with some of the more challenging aspects is great news indeed.

New Relief for Sjögren's Syndrome

Sjögren's syndrome is another mysterious medical problem that primarily affects women. It is characterized by dryness in the mouth, the eyes, and sometimes the nose. This puzzling symptom also stumped the medical profession for years until it was finally recognized as another autoimmune disease.

Sjögren's syndrome resembles fibromyalgia in a number of ways. It too causes pain in the connective tissue, tender points, and soreness; sleep disorders are also a common complaint. And because the mouth becomes so dry, dental problems, including the loss of teeth, are also associated with it.

In addition to having a name that is difficult to spell and pronounce, Sjögren's syndrome is as misunderstood and underreported as fibromyalgia once was. Again, it is a problem that strikes women—particularly older women, although more and more it is being found in women of all ages. Some people with AIDS have it, and it is often associated with lupus.

In Sjögren's, the cells are hyperactive, as they are in many autoimmune diseases. However, with Sjögren's, they are hyperactive precisely when they should be calming down. As a result, sufferers rarely attain the deep sleep on the cellular level that spells real rest.

Until now, there was no medication available to ease the pain arising from Sjögren's syndrome. SAM-e is one of the few treatments that can help. One of my patients, a fifty-nine-year-old woman who has been struggling for many years with Sjögren's, began taking it a while back. Her relief was so dramatic that she's been willing to pay the high cost of bringing it in from Europe—and to ration it to herself to make her small supplies last longer. She never knew when she'd be able to get it again. Now that SAM-e is so easily available in this country, she and the millions of others suffering from Sjögren's syndrome in the United States may find much-needed relief.

More Ways to Help Yourself

SAM-e may help to relieve the pain and depression symptoms of both fibromyalgia and Sjögren's syndrome, but you need to incorporate some changes in your lifestyle to enhance its effectiveness. Most physicians now agree that the approach to treating these conditions must be multidisciplinary. In plain English, that means it requires emphasis on the whole person, mind and body, treating both in harmony with each other. Pay particular attention to Chapters 7 and 8; they can be of great help to you. Here are some other tips that can ease your symptoms.

MASSAGE

A regular series of massages can tremendously ease the muscle pain that accompanies fibromyalgia. During a flare-up of fibromyalgia, the muscles feel like wood or like cellophane crackling under the fingers of the massage therapist. When the patient is getting better, the muscles have a healthier consistency, more like a peeled orange. Massage works to relax the muscles and can bring temporary relief. Such temporary relief on a regular basis can make a world of difference to someone living with fibromyalgia.

If massages are too expensive in your area, consider asking family members or friends who might be interested in massage to learn some basic techniques. Perhaps this new knowledge will lead them to a new interest or career. In the meantime, they can practice on you.

Along with massage, application of heat via a heating pad, hot-water bottle, or whirlpool may ease the soreness. Trying all of these approaches from time to time is certainly worthwhile to see what works for you.

STRETCHING, YOGA, AND ENERGY WORK

Regular stretching is important for everyone, but it is particularly important for people with fibromyalgia. Longer muscles are stronger muscles. Even a little bit of stretching will make you feel better, lengthening muscles that may have become shortened due to lack of exercise and the tension that comes from soreness and pain.

Of course you know how to stretch, but it's a good idea to adopt some specific stretching exercises so that you derive the benefits without straining. Many stretching exercises also contribute to greater flexibility in the joints. All of this helps to reduce the pain associated with fibromyalgia. Just a few minutes of stretching a day will attune you to your own body in a new way.

Combine conscious breathing with your stretching and you're on your way to practicing Yoga, the ancient science of uniting the body with the breath and the spirit. Take a moment now to understand how profoundly simple and beneficial this can be.

Sit up straight in a chair with your shoulders down and back and your chin parallel to the floor. Your arms are dangling at your sides. Now inhale, and as you inhale, lift both arms up to shoulder height. Exhale and feel your shoulders settle into place. Inhale and feel the energy flowing through your arms out toward your fingertips. Close your eyes if you are at ease with that and focus your mind on the breath and on the energy in your arms. Continue as long as you're comfortable holding your arms outstretched, breathing in, breathing out. When you're ready, exhale as you slowly lower your arms back to your lap. Sit for another moment and feel the effects. This exercise is a taste of Yoga.

If you find that you like the feeling you get, look for a Yoga class in your area. They are given in so many places these days—health clubs, community centers, health centers, schools, and more. Tell the instructor you are looking for the gentlest approach. Remember there is no competition in Yoga. Sitting or lying in a class and choosing which postures you will participate in is the best way to honor the Yogic principle that the inner teacher is the best guide.

T'ai Chi is an ancient martial art based upon Taoist philosophy. The best-known form of T'ai Chi involves a series of slow, continuous movements executed in a graceful manner while maintaining a straight and up-right posture with the weight of the body on the legs. However, the core of T'ai Chi is learning to circulate energy through the channels or meridians of the body and harmonizing that balance with the changes of the seasons. Try a T'ai Chi class to see if it is helpful.

REGULAR AEROBIC EXERCISE

Even if you start with only five minutes of exercise and increase that very gradually, you'll be doing your-self a world of good. Soon you'll find the benefits outweighing the muscle soreness. For some of you, a five-minute walk may seem daunting at first. Others may wonder what good a mere five minutes can do you. The answer is, it's a first step. If you add one minute whenever you feel you can, within a short pe-riod of time you'll be doing more. But don't go too fast or too far too quickly. You know that your fitness level is lower as a result of fibromyalgia. Increase it gradu-ally, remembering the old adage that slow and steady wins the race.

Any aerobic exercise increases circulation within the muscles, contributing to a reduction in pain. With SAM-e helping to further reduce the muscle soreness and with a nice hot bath or shower after your walk, you'll feel dramatically better.

Swimming in particular is beneficial, especially if you have injuries, are overweight, or are sensitive to putting too much stress on your joints.

One of the best side effects of any aerobic exercise is that it helps you to sleep better, especially if you do it earlier in the day and not right before bedtime. With more refreshing sleep, everything in life looks and feels better to you, increasing the chances you'll be able to do even more aerobic exercise as time goes on.

RELAXATION AND STRESS REDUCTION

Reducing stress and taking time to simply relax is one of the best prescriptions for just about anything that ails you. We went into detail about specific stress-reduction techniques in Chapter 8. A chronic illness like fibromyalgia can be very stressful. Learning to let go can be every bit as important as taking your daily dose of SAM-e. Read over Chapter 8 and pick the de-stressing techniques that work best for you.

DIETARY DOS AND -DON'TS

- Many people with fibromyalgia have sensitivities to foods. A proper nutritional program is key to making sure the body is well fed and cared for. Today there are many ways to eat well without spending hours on food preparation. Trial and error will tell you which foods your body can use and which to avoid.
- Caffeine, alcohol, and nicotine contribute nothing to the body's health. In fact, they wreak havoc with sleep patterns. Energy levels rise and fall constantly

with these substances. Eliminating or curtailing them is your best bet.

- A mix of high-quality protein, certain types of fat, and slow-burning carbohydrates will give you the nutritional support you need to deal with fibromyalgia, Sjögren's, and the accompanying depression. Stay away from refined sugar and foods with quick-burning carbohydrates, like white bread, bagels, white rice, pasta, cake, and cookies. And let's stop being so afraid of fat. As outlined in Chapter 7, not all fats are bad and fat is crucial to many body functions.

Assemble Your Team

It may well take a team of knowledgeable and caring professionals to get you through the difficulties of fibromyalgia, precisely because it is so multifaceted. Your medical doctor can supervise your tests, medications, and general physical health. A nutritionist may be needed to devise—and sometimes supervise—the eating plan that will make sense for you. A physical therapist can help you design an exercise program with several options for different days and levels of comfort—an approach that will provide enough fitness without adding to your stress.

Psychological counseling and a strong support network will ease the difficulties of coping. Don't be afraid to seek and ask for help.

11

Getting Healthy
with SAM-e

Although this book has focused primarily on SAM-e's remarkable ability to heal depression quickly, safely, and with minimal side effects, we would be remiss if we did not also review several more of its other unique benefits. In addition to being one of the best antidepressants to date, we have seen that SAM-e is a valuable treatment for fibromyalgia, and may even help to protect against heart disease by controlling homocysteine. As we have also noted, it is an excellent treatment for arthritis and liver ailments. And research suggests it may be a potent weapon against brain aging.

It may seem odd that one natural substance can do so much, but given the fact that SAM-e is involved in three major pathways (trans-sulfuration, transmethylation, and transaminopropylation) affecting a vast array of important biological reactions in the body, it is not surprising that it impacts so many different systems.

As described more fully in Chapter 3, SAM-e is a critical player in a process called methylation, a term for an essential chemical pathway in the body. Methylation entails the passing of a methyl group—one carbon and three hydrogen atoms—from one molecule to another. It is a trigger for more than thirty-five methylation reactions, affecting nearly all of the trillions of cells in the body. SAM-e can be powerful medicine.

SAM-e: A New Treatment for Osteoarthritis

Arthritis is a general term for more than a hundred different diseases that involve inflammation of the joints. More than 50 million people in the United States suffer from some form of arthritis. Arthritis can be caused by many unrelated factors, including an autoimmune disorder, injury, Lyme disease, and even gout. The most common form is osteoarthritis, also known as "wear and tear" arthritis.

Osteoarthritis is a degenerative disease caused by the destruction of articular cartilage, the unique substance that lines the joints and prevents bones from grinding against each other. This thin, smooth, resilient lining of cartilage allows the joints to move in a fluid fashion and protects the bone from excessive force and wear. As the cartilage gets worn down, the bones become more exposed, sometimes even rubbing against each other, resulting in pain, stiffness, and swelling. As the joint space narrows, the destruction worsens, and the joint lays down spurs of bone called osteophytes. While the osteophytes provide some stability by filling in the empty space, they make the joints feel stiff and creaky, and eventually restrict movement and cause severe pain.

Osteoarthritis can strike any joint, but it is more likely to affect the weight-bearing joints of the lower limbs, such as the knees and hips. Frequently used smaller joints like those in the hands are often affected. Symptoms of osteoarthritis include morning stiffness (which usually disappears within half an hour of rising) and pain and swelling of the joints. X-ray studies show that seventy-five percent of all people over fifty-five have some form of osteoarthritis, although not everybody has symptoms.

Despite the fact that arthritis is probably the most common ailment suffered by mankind next to the common cold, we know surprisingly little about it. We observe the destructive effect it has on the body, but we really don't know precisely what triggers it, why it happens, or how to prevent it. There are many theories about what causes arthritis. Some researchers believe it is the result of chronic damage by excess free radicals, those troublesome by-products of energy production. Others feel that the decline in key hormones (such as estrogen, testosterone, and growth hormone) inhibits the body's ability to repair damaged cells, resulting in the destruction of joints. Still others say it is simply the result of constant wear and tear which gradually erodes the cartilage. Whatever the cause may turn out to be, osteoarthritis is generally treated symptomatically.

We use scores of over-the-counter and prescription drugs to reduce the pain, swelling, and inflammation of arthritis. Most of these medications fall into the category of nonsteroidal anti-inflammatory drugs (NSAIDs) such as aspirin, naproxen, and ibuprofen. Unfortunately, there are several side effects associated with NSAIDs. The primary one is gastrointestinal upset, which may lead to internal bleeding and even ulcers. NSAIDs block substances known as prostaglandins. Although prostaglandins may be troublemakers in some parts of the body, they help to protect the stomach lining against irritation. Additionally, some people develop kidney or liver problems from chronic use of NSAIDs. Many people must discontinue NSAIDs because of these serious, potentially life-threatening complications. Eight thousand people in the United States alone die each year as a result of bleeding from NSAIDs. NSAIDs relieve symptoms, but some may actually *accelerate* the destruction of cartilage. In other words, they may actually make the arthritis worse!

Recently, millions of people have turned to an alternative treatment for osteoarthritis, glucosamine sulfate and chrondroitin. Known as the "Arthritis Cure," these two natural substances can effectively relieve pain and inflammation without the problems associated with NSAIDs. But as good as these supplements may be, they are not the final answer.

There is tantalizing evidence that SAM-e may be a more effective arthritis treatment than glucosamine and chondroitin sulfate. It not only relieves pain, swelling, stiffness, and redness, but often *stimulates the regrowth of cartilage and lubricates the joint.* SAM-e works as well as NSAIDs in relieving inflammation and swelling, but without the harmful side effects.

SAM-e is approved for use as an arthritis treatment in Germany and is widely used for this purpose throughout Europe. Scientists are enthusiastic about SAM-e and arthritis because it has the potential to help tackle this common disease in several different ways.

But of course, what's most important to patients is the immediate relief of pain, and SAM-e has passed this test with flying colors. Clinical trials of SAM-e involving more than twenty thousand arthritic patients in Europe have consistently produced excellent results. As noted in an issue of the *American Journal of Medicine* entirely devoted to SAM-e and osteoarthritis (November 20, 1987, Vol. 83, supp. 5A), "From these trials SAM-e appears to be effective in pain relief and remarkably free from serious side effects."

Here is a review of other important studies also reported in this issue:

- In a major clinical trial in Germany involving 20,621 patients with osteoarthritis of the knee, hip, spine, and fingers, participants were given 600mg of SAM-e daily for the first two weeks, 400mg for the second two weeks, and 200mg thereafter. The study lasted eight weeks. Evaluation of the clinical findings revealed that eighty percent of the patients reported reduction in the severity of symptoms in all arthritic sites. When asked to rate the efficacy of SAM-e, the participating physicians (orthopedic surgeons and general practitioners) said that SAM-e was "very good" or "good" in seventy percent of their patients, "moderate" for twenty-one percent and "poor" for nine percent. The rate of adverse side effects was very low. Seventy-five percent of the patients rated SAM-e "good" or "very good" in terms of relieving their symptoms. Not only did the patients do well, but the researchers noted that SAM-e "indicates a very high level of drug safety in the field of antirheumatics."

- The results of a two-year multicenter trial involving ten physicians were reported by Dr. Benno Konig at the Institute of General Medicine, University of Mainz, in Germany, in which 108 patients with osteoarthritis of the knee, hip, and spine were given 600mg of SAM-e daily for two weeks, and then 400mg daily for the rest of the study. Dr. Konig's conclusion was that SAM-e was "effective and well tolerated." More than ninety percent of the physicians and eighty-five percent of the patients rated the efficacy of SAM-e as "very good" or "good." Dr. Konig noted, "The clinical efficacy of treatment with SAM-e was evident in all joints assessed." Typically, patients experienced a major decrease in symptoms by the end of the second week of treatment. Not surprisingly, SAM-e also helped to relieve the depression that often accompanies a chronic illness such as arthritis.

- In another double-blind study, conducted by the University School of Medicine, Orthopedics Clinics, in Milan, Italy, SAM-e was compared to both a placebo and naproxen, a standard NSAID in the treatment of osteoarthritis of the hip, knee, spine, and hand. Some 734 patients participated in the study, which was conducted at thirty-three medical centers. As expected, both naproxen and SAM-e did better than the placebo in relieving symptoms. When SAM-e was compared to naproxen, patients taking 1200mg of SAM-e daily had the same pain relief as those taking 750mg of naproxen. Although naproxen worked somewhat faster, SAM-e achieved the same results with far fewer negative side effects. The researchers noted, "The tolerability of SAM-e was superior to that of naproxen and did not differ from that of placebo. . . . SAM-e, because of its analgesic properties and lack of major side effects, deserves to be ranked among the most adequate drugs for the medical management of osteoarthritis."

- In yet another double-blind, randomized study conducted in Buenos Aires, Argentina, SAM-e was compared to the NSAID piroxicam in the management of knee osteoarthritis. Both SAM-e and piroxicam worked well in relieving pain by the twenty-eighth day, with the piroxicam kicking in a bit earlier. When the medication was discontinued after eighty-four days, the good effects of SAM-e were felt long after the effects of the piroxicam had worn off. Although they are both effective, there are good reasons to choose SAM-e over piroxicam. While piroxicam is an effective drug, like other NSAIDs it can cause serious gastric side effects, and can react poorly with other prescription medications—two problems that don't occur with SAM-e.

SAM-e not only relieves pain but also offers other tangible benefits to arthritis patients that NSAIDs do not.

SAM-e protects cartilage. NSAIDs can relieve pain and inflammation but may wear down cartilage. In contrast, as noted, SAM-e protects cartilage from further destruction and may help to stimulate new growth. Although this information is preliminary, it is compelling enough to report here. Animal studies have shown that SAM-e increases the production of chrondrocytes, the cartilage-producing cells in the joint. In theory, the more chondrocytes you have, the more cartilage your body can produce. In studies of rabbits, SAM-e not only boosted chondrocyte production but also produced thicker cartilage. A new German study suggests that SAM-e is having a similarly positive effect on cartilage production in humans. Fourteen patients with finger osteoarthritis were given 400mg of SAM-e daily, while seven patients used as a control were not given any medication. After three months, all patients were given an MRI to determine the condition of the cartilage in the affected area. Those who had been taking SAM-e showed a small but significant increase in cartilage as compared to those in the control group. Although this is a small study, the good results warrant repeating in a larger group.

But that's not all SAM-e does to preserve joint health. It also helps the joint maintain its flexibility and fluidity. The thin layer of cartilage lining the joint has three components: water, collagen, and large molecules called proteoglycans. Proteoglycans are essential because they hold on to water, which provides cartilage with much of its flexibility. Proteoglycans also play an important role in the synovial fluid, the watery space that lubricates the joint, keeping movements smooth. When a joint becomes arthritic, the proteoglycans begin to break down, causing the joint to become unstable. SAM-e helps to prevent the breakdown of proteoglycans, which in turn keeps the joint functioning normally. It's like putting oil in the Tin Man's joints!

SAM-e protects against free radicals. As you know, SAM-e boosts levels of glutathione, an important antioxidant in the body that protects against free radicals, which can damage joint tissue. In fact, several studies have shown that antioxidants—vitamin E, for example—can help to relieve the severity of arthritis. However, antioxidants alone do not have the same analgesic effect as SAM-e, nor have they been shown to stimulate cartilage regrowth.

SAM-e's ability to boost cartilage production raises an interesting question: Can taking SAM-e early in life protect against getting arthritis down the road? Although this question has never been studied—nor is a long-term clinical trial likely, due to cost and time factors—the answer could very well be yes. Anything that both protects cartilage from free radicals and increases cartilage-producing cells could have a positive, long-lasting effect on joint health.

How to Take SAM-e for Arthritis

If you want to take SAM-e for fast relief of arthritic symptoms, start with 800mg daily for the first two weeks, and then reduce your dose to 400mg daily. This is the dosage used by Dr. Peter Billigman for Olympic athletes in Germany. For older patients or those who may be sensitive to stimulating effects of medicines, I often recommend just 400mg daily from the start. Take half of your dose on an empty stomach about half an hour before breakfast, and the other half on an empty stomach about half an hour before lunch. (For more advice, see Chapter 6.)

When it comes to arthritis, SAM-e does not necessarily work faster than NSAIDs. In fact, many NSAIDs provide more rapid pain relief. However, SAM-e does relieve pain within the first few weeks, and again, unlike NSAIDs, SAM-e does not cause any potentially serious side effects.

Protecting the Liver

A healthy body produces about eight grams of SAM-e a day, and more than half of that amount is synthesized in the liver. There's a good reason why so much SAM-e is concentrated in the liver: SAM-e is vital for a healthy, well-functioning liver. Without adequate amounts of SAM-e, the liver cannot do its job.

The liver, one of the body's largest internal organs, performs many necessary functions. It detoxifies alcohol, drugs, and other poisons naturally found in foods (such as insecticides and preservatives) before they can destroy healthy cells in other parts of the body. It breaks down steroid hormones (such as estrogen and testosterone) and produces clotting factors, blood proteins, and thousands of different enzymes necessary for countless biological reactions. It is crucial to the production of bile, an essential digestive acid. A well-functioning liver is more than key to good health; it is critical for survival.

Under normal circumstances, the liver regenerates itself and produces new cells as old ones wear out. In cases of liver disease, such as hepatitis B or C or alcohol-induced cirrhosis, portions of the liver become hardened and inactive. The liver loses its ability to regrow cells and eventually stops functioning normally.

Studies have shown that in patients with liver disease, SAM-e levels are abnormally low. Patients show a deficiency in the enzyme necessary to convert methionine to SAM-e, leading to a glitch in its production. This can be catastrophic. Without SAM-e, the liver cannot make enough glutathione, the body's primary detoxifying antioxidant. Without glutathione, deadly toxins will begin to build up throughout the body, and that can be fatal.

Not only is SAM-e involved in glutathione production, but there is evidence that it helps to preserve liver health in other ways. As part of the methylation cycle, we have seen that SAM-e is also essential for numerous activities (such as phospholipid methylation and protein methylation) that help maintain cell growth and repair. When SAM-e levels decline, the liver cannot perform these functions as effectively.

SAM-e has been used successfully as a treatment for

liver disease in Italy. Studies have found that SAM-e supplements can undo the breakdown in its production in the liver by normalizing the levels of the key enzyme associated with SAM-e production: SAM-e supplements help the liver to make more SAM-e. As SAM-e levels rise, so do levels of beneficial glutathione.

It comes as no surprise that excess alcohol can be a lethal poison; it accelerates the production of a particularly toxic free radical called acetaldehyde. In most cases, the body can handle a glass or two of wine, but more than that daily for an extended period of time causes liver damage by wiping out its supply of glutathione. It seems that SAM-e not only increases glutathione levels, but it helps to reduce the craving for alcohol. SAM-e also combats the depression that so often accompanies alcohol addiction. Both animal and human studies have confirmed that SAM-e supplementation can halt alcohol-related liver damage, and allow the healing process to begin.

Interferon is a potent drug commonly used to treat hepatitis C. Unfortunately, it has a nasty side effect— it can trigger depression. Because the liver is already under siege, physicians are reluctant to prescribe antidepressants, which must be broken down by the liver. Why put a further load on liver function? This is an area in which I'm beginning to see some results. I've given patients SAM-e in conjunction with interferon to treat hepatitis-related cirrhosis of the liver, and have seen improvements in mood and liver function. For patients with hepatitis, SAM-e can lift the depression that often goes along with the disease, and can possibly accelerate the healing of the liver itself.

SAM-e has also been used to treat intrahepatic cholestasis of pregnancy (a syndrome that mimics a mechanical obstruction of the biliary tract). As noted, estrogen is broken down by the liver. Excess estrogen may induce cholestasis in sensitive women, which is characterized by the accumulation of bile in liver cells and biliary passages. This potentially serious condition can result in premature delivery and harm to the fetus. During pregnancy, physicians are often reluctant to give medication unless it is absolutely necessary, because of potential risks to the fetus. Fortunately, SAM-e has been proven to be an effective treatment for cholestasis, safe for both mother and baby.

SAM-e and the Aging Brain

The rate of depression is two to three times higher among the elderly than in younger populations. Granted, the later decades can be fraught with new problems, losses, and challenges that can trigger depression in even the hardiest people. It is a time when many fall victim to the diseases of aging, when spouses and friends die, and when retirement forces people to reinvent themselves. For many it is a time of tumultuous change, and change, whether it is good or bad, can be stressful.

There are also specific changes in brain chemistry that not only contribute to depression but are responsible for the age-related decline in mental function. For example, by the sixth decade, most people notice a decline in short-term memory. Medical tests can even detect it by age forty! This is such a common occurrence that there's even a name for it—age-associated memory impairment (AAMI). Some people may have difficulty concentrating for long periods of time or learning new tasks.

Why does the brain begin to slow down? In some cases, there is an easy explanation. For example, many drugs commonly prescribed for physical ailments of aging, such as heart disease, may interfere with brain chemistry, resulting in confusion, memory loss, and other symptoms. As discussed in Chapter 7, poor nutrition can result in a deficiency of key vitamins, which could cause confusion, memory loss, and depression. But such simple explanations do not fully explain the phenomenon, which can occur even in the absence of these common culprits.

We don't fully understand what causes brain aging. So far we have a lot of theories and few proven facts. There is a growing consensus among scientists, however, that the same forces that are aging the body are also aging the brain. When it comes to the brain, these forces do their dirty work even faster.

SAM-e may help reverse, and perhaps prevent, some of these destructive changes.

Free Radicals Target the Brain

The brain is the most active organ in the body; it is always hard at work. Every moment, every heartbeat, must first be coordinated by the brain. The brain needs a continuous supply of blood and oxygen to fuel this activity. But, as we have seen, oxygen is a double-edged sword. The more oxygen that's burned for energy, the more free radicals the brain produces. And to make matters worse, the brain is more than fifty percent fat, and fat is particularly vulnerable to free radical attack. Just like the fat in meat, it can go rancid when exposed to oxygen. Free radicals can target the fat in neurons, and neurons produce the neurotransmitters. As more and more neurons are destroyed, production of neurotransmitters declines. This sets the stage for depression and other cognitive problems. Many researchers believe that an excess of free radicals contributes to both Alzheimer's disease and Parkinson's disease.

Recently, there have been many supplements touted as "brain boosters" or "memory cures." These supplements typically fall into three categories. They are either antioxidants, which help control free radicals, or natural boosters of one or more of the neurotransmitters which decline with age, or metabolic boosters of nerve metabolism. SAM-e takes a more sophisticated approach to brain aging: it tackles the problem where it begins, at the cellular level.

SAM-e enables the body to produce more of its free radical scavenger, glutathione. At the same time, it boosts the levels of transmitters involved in mood, memory, and learning. In a sense, SAM-e restores the brain to a more youthful environment. Interestingly, people with Alzheimer's disease have lower-than-normal levels of SAM-e. We're not suggesting that taking SAM-e can prevent or cure Alzheimer's, but by boosting antioxidant levels, it might help maintain a healthier environment in the brain, which could have an effect on Alzheimer's disease. When it comes to Alzheimer's, there are still many more questions than answers.

SAM-e may attack the problem of brain aging in other important ways. It can increase the phosphatidylcholine content of the nerve cell membrane.

SAM-e Controls Homocysteine

As we discussed earlier, too much homocysteine can be dangerous to every organ in the body, especially the brain. High levels of this amino acid are associated with depression and dementia. Homocysteine not only is toxic to the nerve cells in the brain, but also destroys the cells that line the arteries. This diminishes the delivery of blood and oxygen throughout the body, and leads to coronary artery disease. A working brain needs to have a constant supply of blood and oxygen. If the circulation is diminished, the brain will be forced to function at less than optimal levels.

SAM-e, as we demonstrated in Chapter 3, is critical for the homocysteine cycle. The folic acid supplement we recommend in Chapter 7 helps SAM-e keep homocysteine tightly controlled to prevent the deadly process that can lead to serious cognitive problems.

SAM-e Rejuvenates Receptors

There's yet another way, also noted in Chapter 3, that SAM-e can help keep our brain cells functioning at higher levels—by keeping them more flexible and resilient. Every cell in the body is encased in a protective cell membrane—the gatekeeper of the cell. A healthy cell membrane allows the easy passage of nutrients into the cell, and ushers waste products out. As we age, our cell membranes become rigid, no longer functioning as well as flexible young ones.

Cell membranes are made of substances called phospholipids. Phospholipids are kept in steady supply by a process called phospholipid methylation, which declines as we age. Phospholipid methylation is one of the methylation cycles that depend on SAM-e.

Animal studies strongly suggest that SAM-e has a very positive effect on brain cells in older animals. Rats experience many of the same age-related biochemical changes that occur in humans. Not only do their cell membranes lose the ability to freely exchange chemicals, but they also lose significant numbers of receptors,

the important structures that translate chemical messages into and out of the cell. In one experiment, rats
well into middle age were given SAM-e for thirty days.
At the end of the study, researchers examined the brain
cell membranes in the hippocampus (the memory center of the brain). They found that the membranes had
been restored to a more youthful state—they did
not have the telltale rigidity of an old cell. And the
SAM-e–treated rats had grown *new* receptors, those involved in memory and learning. Follow-up studies
have shown that if young rats are given SAM-e, it can
protect against the age-related loss of these important
receptors. Does this mean that SAM-e will help humans stay smarter and sharper throughout old age? It's
premature to say yes, but there is good reason to think
that it will have a positive effect.

Treating Parkinson's Disease

Parkinson's disease is a degenerative neurological disorder known for its characteristic tremors. Its slow,
jerky movements can become severe enough to hamper
mobility. Parkinson's is caused by the malfunctioning
of a particular group of brain cells called the substan-
tia nigra, which releases the neurotransmitter dopamine.

Parkinson's affects primarily the elderly, but in rare
cases can strike people in their twenties. About forty
percent of people with Parkinson's also suffer from de-

pression. They don't necessarily exhibit the classic symptoms of depression. Instead, they sink into a state of hopelessness and despair.

There is no cure for Parkinson's. As with other degenerative diseases, symptoms can worsen over time. Sinemet is the drug most widely prescribed for the treatment of Parkinson's. It is a combination of levodopa (better known as L-dopa) and carbidopa, which slows the breakdown of L-dopa. Although L-dopa can help to relieve the tremors and involuntary muscle movements, it does not work for everyone. And if it does work, eventually the effectiveness tapers off. There's another problem with L-dopa. It depletes SAM-e levels, which may make Parkinson's sufferers even more vulnerable to depression. However, SAM-e supplements can help reverse this depression without interfering with the ability of L-dopa to treat Parkinson's symptoms. A 1990 study published in *Current Therapeutic Research* (Vol. 48, No. 1) reported that after two weeks of treatment with SAM-e, seventy-two percent of Parkinson's patients showed improvement in mood, versus only thirty percent of those who took a placebo.

Terry and I recently participated in a study on the treatment of SAM-e for depression in Parkinson's disease in the department of neurology at New York's Beth Israel Medical Center. Our coinvestigators included Drs. J. D. Rogers and A. DiRocco, two neurologists. Eight patients completed the trial, which included a daily dose of SAM-e that began at 800mg and was gradually raised to as much as 3300mg. Patients were given a standard depression-rating test (the Hamilton Rating Scale) before and after treatment. On this test, a score of 18 is considered severe depression. For our patients, the mean Hamilton score before treatment with SAM-e was 28.3. After two months on SAM-e, the mean Hamilton score fell to 8—not within the depressed range at all! Presenting our findings at the XIII International Congress on Parkinson's Disease in Vancouver, we concluded, "SAM-e may be a safe and effective agent for the treatment of depression in Parkinson's disease. Further controlled studies are necessary to evaluate its efficacy and safety in Parkinson's disease."

In my practice, I have used SAM-e for patients with Parkinson's with equally good results. Although SAM-e is not a cure, my clinical experience shows that it does improve the depression of Parkinson's while relieving some of the muscle spasms and tremors. Moreover, SAM-e improves the response of patients to their L-dopa, meaning that they can stay on this beneficial drug for longer periods with better response. Since SAM-e boosts levels of dopamine, the neurotransmitter most affected by Parkinson's, it just may be an important development in Parkinson's disease treatment. For some people, SAM-e works remarkably well. As one patient, a seventy-two-year-old recently diagnosed with Parkinson's put it, "It lifts you up, you feel more positive. I'm sleeping better, I'm eating better, I have more energy, and I feel more in control."

If you have Parkinson's disease, talk with your doctor about whether you should take SAM-e.

SAM-e is powerful medicine against depression. It works as well as any prescription antidepressant and better than most. Not only that, SAM-e brings relief in a fraction of the time while causing no notable side effects.

That would be enough.

But, even better, SAM-e is not a drug. It's a substance already found in our bodies, a molecule essential for life. Restoring it to optimal levels can produce major health benefits.

No one with depression should have to suffer in silence. No one with depression should believe that depression is an inevitable way of life. For the majority of you, depression can be reduced to a bad memory.

Throughout this book, we have shown you how you can stop your depression, quickly and effectively. We wrote this book to encourage and empower you to get help for your depression. It is our hope that many people whose depression has gone untreated, who have feared going to a psychiatrist, or who have been reluctant to admit to feeling low will feel free to seek help. Maybe those of you who don't think of yourselves as depressed but for whom life could be better—the millions of you in the gray zone—will also gain relief. We hope that many of you who have sought help and found prescription drugs intolerable or found yourselves inadequately treated can now have your depression lifted.

SAM-e is a solid first step on the road to recovery. For most of you, it will work remarkably fast and cause none of the negative side effects associated with other antidepressants. You may also enjoy the additional benefits we have described here.

Yet SAM-e needs some help from you. To stay depression-free, you may need to make significant changes in your lifestyle or add counseling or psychotherapy to your SAM-e regimen.

Now the tools to stop depression are in your hands. Use them.

A Letter to Physicians

Dear Colleagues:

Stop Depression Now is geared toward the lay public. However, beyond that, Teodoro Bottiglieri and I hope this book will be a useful introduction to the potential benefits of SAM-e for clinicians and researchers alike. I'd like to draw your attention to the list of scientific references immediately following this letter. SAM-e has undergone rigorous scientific scrutiny, and as you can see, the findings of these first-class studies have been published in some of the world's premier peer-reviewed journals.

Since beginning work on *Stop Depression Now,* I have heard a number of questions from other medical professionals. I'd like to take the opportunity to answer those questions now.

If SAM-e is so good, why haven't we heard about it?

As we are all too well aware, the financial pressures and time constraints on today's physicians are intense. Hour upon hour of precious office time is spent filling out insurance forms, making referrals, and advocating for our patients' rights to medical coverage. Moreover, information overload has not spared our profession. The sheer volume of good research being done and published worldwide makes it nearly impossible to stay as current in our fields as we ought to.

In this fog of knowledge, we pay attention to the information most clearly delineated. Like it or not, that information comes most often from the pharmaceutical companies. Only they can afford to disseminate knowledge with the volume and frequency necessary to cut through everything else. This has been going on for a while now, and busy physicians sometimes lose sight of the fact that pharmaceutical companies and their representatives are not our only source of new information. Natural, nonpatented products have little chance of catching the attention of the medical community in this environment. Consequently, we most often learn of anything natural from our patients—not vice versa.

There is another factor at work here as well. Namely, it takes an awfully long time for treatments, especially foreign ones, to gain acceptance in the United States. Lithium, for example, was first used in Australia to treat bipolar disorder in 1949. It was not embraced for regular use here until 1974—

twenty-five years later. In another case, I began speaking about Depakote (valproic acid) as a treatment for bipolar disorder in 1979, more than fifteen years before its widespread use in 1996. Similarly, SAM-e was first studied in 1972. Now, twenty-seven years later, it is making its debut on the American consciousness.

Can one substance realistically do all these things? It seems too good to be true.

The answer is a resounding *yes.* As we have said throughout *Stop Depression Now,* SAM-e is a natural substance already found in our bodies. It is crucial for three major biochemical pathways and lies at the center of thirty-five important chemical reactions in the body. Frankly, it would be surprising if SAM-e did *not* affect so many systems.

To fully understand why SAM-e is so varied in its effects, you must grasp its biochemistry. I urge you to review the work of my coauthor, Teodoro Bottiglieri, and the other biochemists who have studied this molecule. At the risk of glossing too lightly over their work, I can outline in broad strokes the essential metabolic pathways involving SAM-e.

As you know, SAM-e is a methyl donor and that accounts for its broad range of therapeutic action. The three main metabolic pathways involving SAM-e are transmethylation, trans-sulfuration, and trans-aminopropylation. Transmethylation, the pathway we are most concerned with in this book, accounts for SAM-e's antidepressant action. However, trans-methylation also impacts on SAM-e's analgesic and anti-inflammatory activities. Transaminopropy-lation also contributes to SAM-e's analgesic and anti-inflammatory action while stimulating proteoglycan synthesis and protecting the gastrointestinal tract lining—two results shared by the trans-sulfuration pathway.

How can you let patients treat themselves?

Depression is underdiagnosed and undertreated in America. For numerous people, this will be the first opportunity they have had to get help. Since SAM-e is available over the counter, Teodoro Bottiglieri and I felt that a popular book would be the best way to ed-ucate the public. After all, the power to use SAM-e is in their hands—not ours.

SAM-e is easily available, and it works. People will find it, and they will use it. They should know how.

What about the use of SAM-e with other antidepressants?

I have used SAM-e at 400mg or higher orally with nearly every antidepressant available, with the excep-tion of MAO inhibitors. (SAM-e has not been tested for use with MAO inhibitors, and this combination should be avoided pending further study.) The result of this use of SAM-e with other antidepressants has been an acceleration and enhancement of antidepressant re-sponse. For an excellent clinical study on this phenomenon, I call your attention to Berlanga et al, *Psychiatry Res* 1992, 44: 257–62.

Although SAM-e has been used in pregnant women with no ill effects, more studies are needed to establish its safety in pregnant and nursing women.

I hope this book inspires you to investigate the therapeutic potential of SAM-e for your patients. I hope it will stimulate more research about SAM-e, as is being done by my neurologist colleagues Dr. Alex DiRocco and Dr. John Rogers of the Beth Israel–Albert Einstein College of Medicine. In addition, I believe that more research exploring the interface between essential nutrients and antidepressants would lead to many new and worthwhile treatments.

RICHARD BROWN, M.D.
April 5, 1999

Bibliography

SAM-E AND DEPRESSION

Agnoli, A.; Andreoli, V.; Casacchia, M.; et al. "Effect of S-adenosylmethionine upon depressive symptoms." *Journal of Psychiatry Research* 1976, 13: 43–54.

Agricola, R.; Dalla Verde, G.; Urani, R.; et al. "S-adenosyl-L-methionine in the treatment of major depression complicating chronic alcoholism." *Current Therapeutic Research* 1994, 55: 83–92.

Andreoli, V. M.; Maffei, F.; and Tonon, G. C. "S-adenosyl-L-methionine (SAMe) blood levels in schizophrenia and depression." *Transmethylation and the Central Nervous System,* New York: Springer Verlag, 1978, 147–50.

Baldessarini, R. "Neuropharmacology of S-adenosyl-L-methionine." *American Journal of Medicine,* November 1987, 83 (5A): 95–103.

Bell, K. M.; Plon, L.; Bunney, W. E.; and Potkin, S. G. "S-adenosylmethionine treatment of depression: a controlled clinical trial." *American Journal of Psychiatry* 1988, 145: 1110–14.

Berlanga, C.; Ortega-Soto, H. A.; Ontiveros, M.; and Senties, H. "Efficacy of S-adenosyl-L-methionine in speeding the onset of action of imipramine." *Journal of Psychiatry Research,* December 1992, 44 (3): 257–62.

Bottiglieri, T. "Ademetionine (S-adenosylmethionine) neuropharmacology: implications for drug therapies in psychiatric and neurological disorders." *Expert Opinion in Investigational Drugs* 1997, 6: 417–26.

Bottiglieri, T.; Chary, T. K. N.; Laundy, M.; Carney, M. W. P.; Godfrey, P.; Toone, B. K.; and Reynolds, E. H. "Transmethylation and Depression." *Alabama Journal of Medical Science* 1988, 25: 296–300.

Bottiglieri, T., Godfrey, P., Flyno, T., et al. "Cerebrospinal fluid S-adenosylmethionine in depression and dementia: effects of treatment with parenteral and oral S-adenosylmethionine." *Journal of Neurology, Neurosurgery & Psychiatry* 1990, 53 (12): 1096–98.

Bottiglieri, T., and Hyland, K. "S-adenosylmethionine levels in psychiatric and neurological disorders: a review." *Acta Scandinavica Neurologica* 1994, 89 (154): 19–26.

Bottiglieri, T.; Laundy, M.; Martin, R.; Carney, M. W. P.; Nissenbaum, H.; Toone, B. K.; Johnson, A. L.; and Reynolds, E. H. "S-adenosylmethionine influences monoamine metabolism." *Lancet* 1984, 2: 224.

Bressa, G. M. "S-adenosyl-L-methionine (SAMe) as antidepressant: meta-analysis of clinical studies." *Acta Scandinavica Neurologica* 1994, 89(154): 7–14.

Carney, M. W. P.; Chary, T.K.N.; Bottiglieri, T.; et al. "Switch mechanism in affective illness and oral S-adenosylmethionine (SAM)." *British Journal of Psychiatry* 1987; 150: 724–725.

Cerutti, R.; Sichel, M. P.; Perin, M.; Grussu, P.; and Zulian, O. "Psychological distress during puerperium: a novel therapeutic approach using S-adenosylmethionine." *Current Therapeutic Research* 1993, 53: 707–16.

Crellin, R.; Bottiglieri, T.; and Reynolds, E. H. "Folates and psychiatric disorders. *Drugs* 1993, 45: 623–36.

Curcio, M.; Catto, E.; Stramentinoli, G.; and Algeri, S. "Effect of SAMe on 5HT metabolism in rat brain." *Progress in Neuropsychopharmacology* 1978, 2: 65–71.

Czyrak, A.; Rogoz, Z.; Skuza, G.; Zajaczkowski, W.; and Maj, J. "Antidepressant activity of S-adenosylmethionine in mice and rats." *Journal of Basic Clinical Physiological Pharmacology* 1992, 3: 1–17.

De Leo, D. "S-adenosylmethionine as an antidepressant—a double-blind trial versus placebo." *Current Therapeutic Research* 1987, 7: 254–57.

De Vanna, M., and Rigamonti, R. "Oral S-adenosylmethionine in depression." *Current Therapeutic Research* 1992, 52: 478–85.

Fava, M.; Rosenbaum, J. F.; MacLaughlin, R.; et al. "Neuroendocrine effects of S-adenosyl-L-methionine, a novel putative antidepressant." *Journal of Psychiatry Research* 1990, 24 (2): 177–84.

Fava, M.; Fiannelli, A.; Rapisarda, V.; et al. "Rapidity of onset of the antidepressant effect of parenteral S-adenosyl-L-methionine." *Journal of Psychiatry Research,* April 1995, 56 (3): 295–97.

Fava, M.; Borus, J. S.; Alpert, J. E.; Nierenberg, A.; Rosenbaum, J. F.; and Bottiglieri, T. "Folate, B_{12} and homocysteine in major depression. *American Journal of Psychiatry* 1997, 154: 426–28.

Janicak, P. G.; Lipinski, J. D.; Comaty, J. E.; Waternaux, C.; Cohen, B.; Altman, E.; and Sharma, R. P. "S-adenosylmethionine, a literature review and preliminary report." *Alabama Journal of Medical Science* 1988, 25: 306–13.

Kagan, B.; Sultzer, D. L.; Rosenlicht, N.; and Gerner, R. H. "Oral S-adenosylmethionine in depression: a randomized, double-blind, placebo-controlled trial." *American Journal of Psychiatry* 1990, 147: 591–95.

Kufferle, B., and Grunberger, J. "Early clinical double-blind study with S-adenosyl-L-methionine: a new potential antidepressant," in: Costa, E., and Racagni, G., eds.: *Typical and Atypical Antidepressants: Clinical practice.* New York: Raven Press, 1982: 175–80.

Lipinski, J. F.; Cohen, B. M.; Frankenburg, F.; et al. "An open trial of S-adenosylmethionine for treatment of depression." *American Journal of Psychiatry* 1984, 141: 448–50.

Mantero, P.; Pastorino, P.; Carolei, A.; et al. "Controlled double-blind study (SAM-e imipramine) in depressive syndromes [in Italian]." *Minerva Medica* 1975, 66: 4098–4101.

Miccoli, L.; Porro, V.; and Bertolino, A. "Comparison between the antidepressant activity of S-adenosyl-L-methionine

(SAMe) and that of some tricyclic drugs." *Acta Neurologica* 1978, 33: 243–55.

Monaco, P., and Quattrocchi, F. "Study of the antidepressive effects of a biological transmethylating agent (S-adenosylmethionine of SAM) [in Italian]." *Rivista di Neurologia,* November-December 1979, 49 (6): 417–39.

Muscettola, G.; Galzenati, M.; and Balbi, A. "SAMe versus placebo: a double-blind comparison in major depressive disorders," in: Costa, E., and Racagni, G., eds.: *Typical and Atypical Antidepressants: Clinical Practice.* New York: Raven Press, 1982: 151–56.

Otero-Losado, M. E., and Rubio, M. C. "Acute changes in 5HT metabolism after S-adenosylmethionine administration." *General Pharmacology* 1989, 20: 403–6.

Otero-Losado, M. E., and Rubio, M. C. "Acute effects of S-adenosyl-L-methionine on catecholaminergic central function." *European Journal of Pharmacology* 1989, 163: 353–56.

Pezzoli, C.; Galli-Kienle, M.; and Stramentinoli, G. "Lack of Mutagenic Activity of Ademetionine in Vitro and in Vivo." *Arzneimittel-Forschung,* July 1987, 37 (7): 826–29.

Pinzello, A., and Andreoli, V. "Le transmetilazioni SAM-e dipendenti nelle sidromi depressive. Valutazione dell-effetto terapeutico dell S-adenosyl-L-methionina con la scala de Hamilton." *Quad Ter Sper Suppl Bioch Biol Sper* 1972, X/2: 3–11.

Rakasz, E.; Sugar, J.; and Csuka, O. "Modulation of Cytosine Arabinoside-Induced Proliferation Inhibition by Exogenous Adenosylmethionine." *Cancer Chemotherapy & Pharmacology* 1991, 28 (5): 484–86.

Rocco, P. L. "Major depression complicating medical illness: Utility of S-adenosyl-L-methionine." *Neuropharmacology* 1994, 10 (2): 99.

Salmaggi, P.; Bressa, G. M.; Nicchia, G.; Coniglio, M.; La Greca, P.; and Le Grazie, C. "Double-blind, placebo-controlled study of S-adenosylmethionine in depressed post-menopausal women." *Psychotherapy and Psychosomatics* 1993, 59: 34–40.

Salvadorini, F.; Galeone, F.; Saba, P.; et al. "Evaluation of S-adenosylmethionine (SAMe) effectiveness on depression." *Current Therapeutic Research* 1980, 20: 908–18.

Scaggion, G.; Baldan, L.; and Domanin, S.; et al "Antidepressive action of S-adenosylmethionine compared to nomifensine maleate [in Italian]." *Minerva Psichiatria* 1982, 23: 93–97.

Scarzella, R., and Appiotti, A. "A double-blind clinical comparison of SAMe vs. clomipramine in depressive disorders [in Italian]." *Riv Sper Freniatr* 1978, 102: 359–65.

Spillmann, M., and Fava, M. "S-adenosylmethionine in psychiatric disorders—historical perspective and current aspects." *CNS Drugs* 1996, 6: 416–25.

Stramentinoli, G. "S-Adenosylmethionine: Pharmacokinetics and Pharmacodynamics." *American Journal of Medicine,* November 1987, 83 (5A): 35–42.

Taylor, K. M., and Randall, P. K. "Depletion of S-adenosyl-L-methionine in mouse brain by antidepressive drugs." *Journal of Pharmacology Experimental Therapeutics* 1975, 94: 303–10.

Torta, R.; Zanalda, E.; Rocca, P.; et al. "Inhibitory activity of S-adenosyl-L-methionine on serum gamma-glutamyltranspeptidase increase induced by psychodrugs and anti-convulsants." *Current Therapeutic Research* 1988, 44: 144–59.

SAM-E AND ARTHRITIS

Adams, M. E. "Cartilage Research and Treatment of Osteoarthritis." *Current Opinion on Rheumatology,* August 1992, 4 (4): 552–59.

Barcelo, H. A.; Weimeyer, J. C.; Sagasta, C. I.; et al. "Effects of S-Adenosylmethionine on Experimental Arthritis in Rabbits." *American Journal of Medicine,* November 1987, 83 (5A): 55–59.

Barcelo, H. A.; Weimeyer, J. C.; Sagasta, C. I.; et al. "Experimental Osteoarthritis and Its Course When Treated with S-Adenosyl-L-Methionine." *Revista Clínica Española,* June 1990, 187 (2): 74–78.

Berger, R., and Nowak, H. "A New Medical Approach to the Treatment of Osteoarthritis. Report of an Open Phase IV Study with Ademetionine (Gumbarat)." *American Journal of Medicine,* November 1987, 83 (5A): 840–48.

Bradley, J. D.; Flusser, D.; Katz, B. P.; et al. "A Randomized, Double-Blind, Placebo-Controlled Trial of Intravenous Loading with S-Adenosylmethionine (SAM) Followed by Oral SAM Therapy in Patients with Knee Osteoarthritis." *Journal of Rheumatology* 1994, 21 (5): 905–1.

Caruso, I., and Pietrograde, V. "Italian Double-Blind Multicenter Study Comparing S-Adenosylmethionine, Naproxen, and Placebo in the Treatment of Degenerative Joint Disease." *American Journal of Medicine,* November 1987, 83 (5A): 66–71.

Di Padova, C. "S-Adenosylmethionine in the Treatment of Osteoarthritis: Review of the Clinical Studies." *American Journal of Medicine,* November 1987, 83 (5A): 60–65.

Domljan, Z.; Vrbovac, B.; Durrigl, T.; et al. "A Double-Blind Trial of Ademetionine vs. Naproxen in Activated Gonarthritis." *International Journal of Clinical Pharmacology, Therapy & Toxicology,* July 1989, 27 (7): 329–33.

Glorioso, S.; Todesco, S.; Mazzi, A.; et al. "Double-Blind Multicentre Study of the Activity of S-Adenosylmethionine in Hip and Knee Osteoarthritis." *International Journal of Clinical Pharmacology Research* 1985, 5 (1): 39–49.

Gualano, M.; Stramentinoli, G.; and Berti, F. "Anti-inflammatory activity of S-adenosylmethionine: interference with the eicosanoid system," *Pharmacological Research Communications* 1983, 15: 683–96.

Harmand, M. F.; Vilamitjana, J.; Maloche, E.; et al. "Effects of S-Adenosylmethionine on Human Articular Chondrocyte Differentiation: An in Vitro Study." *American Journal of Medicine,* November 1987, 83 (5A): 48–54.

Kalbhen, D. A., and Jansen, G. "Pharmacologic Studies on the Antidegenerative Effects of Ademetionine in Experimental Arthritis in Animals." *Arzneimittel-Forschung,* September 1990, 40 (9): 1017–21.

Konig, B. "A Long-Term (Two Years) Clinical Trial with S-Adenosylmethionine for the Treatment of Osteoarthritis." *American Journal of Medicine,* November 1987, 83 (5A): 89–94.

Maccagno, A.; DiGiorgio, E. E.; Caston, O. L.; and Sagasta, C. L. "Double-Blind Controlled Clinical Trial of Oral S-Adenosylmethionine versus Piroxicam in Knee Osteoarthritis." *American Journal of Medicine,* November 1987, 83 (5A): 72–77.

Manicourt, D. H.; Druetz-Van Egeren, A.; Haazen, L.; et al. "Effects of Tenoxican and Aspirin on the Metabolism of Proteoglycans and Hyaluronan in Normal and Osteoarthritic Human Articular Cartilage." *British Journal of Pharmacology,* December 1994, 113 (4): 1113–20.

Marcolongo, R.; Giordano, N.; Colombo, B.; et al. "Double-blind multicentre study of the activity of S-adenosyl-methionine in hip and knee osteoarthritis." *Current Therapeutic Research* 1985, 37: 82–94.

Montrone, F.; Fumagali, M.; Sarzi-Puttini, P.; et al. "Double-blind study of S-adenosyl-methionine versus placebo in hip and knee arthrosis." *Clinical Rheumatology,* December 1985, 4 (4): 484–85.

Muller-Fassbender, H. "Double-Blind Clinical Trial of S-Adenosylmethionine Versus Ibuprofen in the Treatment of Osteoarthritis." *American Journal of Medicine,* November 1987, 83 (5A): 81–3.

Polli, E.; Cortellaro, M.; Patrini, L.; et al. "Pharmacological and Clinical Aspects of S-Adenosylmethionine (SAMe) in Primary Degenerative Arthropathy (Osteoarthritis)." *Minerva Medica,* December 1975, 66 (83): 4443–59.

Reichelt, A.; Forster, K.; Fischer, M.; et al. "Efficacy and Safety of Intramuscular Glucosamine Sulfate in Osteoarthritis of the Knee: A Randomized, Placebo-Controlled, Double-Blind Study." *Arzneimittel-Forschung,* January 1994, 44 (1): 75–80.

Schumacher, H. R.; Moskowitz, R. W.; and Fassbender, H. G.

"Osteoarthritis: The Clinical Picture, Pathogenesis and Management with Studies on a New Therapeutic Agent, S-adenosylmethionine." *American Journal of Medicine,* November 1987, 83 (5A): 1–110.

Setnikar, I. "Antireactive Properties of Chondroprotective Drugs." *International Journal of Tissue Reactions* 1992, 14 (5): 253–61.

Vetter, C. "Double-Blind Comparative Clinical Trial with S-Adenosylmethionine and Indomethacin in the Treatment of Osteoarthritis." *American Journal of Medicine,* November 1987, 83 (5A).

Vignon, E.; Chapuy, M. C.; Arlot, M.; et al. "Study of the Concentration of Glycosaminoglycans in Cartilage from Normal and Osteoarthritic Femoral Head." *Pathologie Biologie,* April 1975, 23 (4): 283–89.

For information on the use of SAM-e for the treatment of arthritis, we refer you to the November 20, 1987, issue of the *American Journal of Medicine* (Volume 83:5A), which was devoted entirely to SAM-e.

SAM-E AND THE AGING BRAIN

Ando, S.; Tanaka, Y.; Ono, Y.; et al. "Incorporation Rate of Gm1 Ganglioside into Mouse Brain Myelin: Effect of Aging Modification by Hormones and Other Compounds." *Advances in Experimental Medicine & Biology* 1984, 174: 241–48.

Bottiglieri, T.; Hyland, K.; and Reynolds, E. H. "The clinical potential of ademethionine (S-adenosylmethionine) in neurological disorders." *Drugs,* August 1994, 48 (2): 137–52.

Carrieri, P. B.; Indaco, A.; Gentile, S.; Troisi, E.; and Campanella, G. "S-adenosylmethionine treatment of depression in patients with Parkinson's disease: a double-blind, crossover study versus placebo." *Current Therapeutic Research* 1990, 48: 154–60.

Cheng, H.; Gomes-Trolin, C.; Aquilonius, S. M.; et al. "Levels of L-methionine S-adenosyltransferase activity in erythrocytes and concentrations of S-adenosylmethionine and S-adenosylhomocysteine in whole blood of patients with Parkinson's disease." *Experimental Neurology* 1997, 145: 580–85.

Cimino, M.; Vantini, G.; Algeri, S.; Curala, G.; Pezzoli, C.; and Stramentinoli, G. "Age-related modification of dopaminergic and beta-adrenergic receptor system: restoration to normal activity by modifying membrane fluidity with S-adenosylmethionine." *Life Sciences* 1984, 34: 2029–39, 41.

Cohen, B. M.; Satlin, A.; and Zubenko, G. S. "S-adenosyl-L-methionine in the treatment of Alzheimer's disease." *Journal of Clinical Psychopharmacology* 1988, 8: 43–47.

Fontanari, D.; Di Palma, C.; Giorgetti, G.; et al. "Effects of S-adenosyl-L-methionine on cognitive and vigilance functions in elderly." *Current Therapeutic Research* 1994, 55(6): 682–89.

Morrison, L. D.; Smith, D. D.; and Kish, S. J. "Brain S-Adenosylmethionine Levels Are Severely Decreased in Alzheimer's Disease." *Journal of Neurochemistry,* September 1996, 57 (3): 1328–31.

Muccioli, G., and Dicardo, R. "S-Adenosyl-L-Methionine Restores Prolactin Receptors in the Aged Rabbit Brain." *European Journal of Pharmacology,* July 1989, 166 (2): 223–30.

Muccioli, G.; Scordamaglia, A.; Bertacco, S.; et al. "Effects of S-adenosylmethionine on brain muscarinic receptors of aged rats." *European Journal of Pharmacology,* November 1992, 227 (3): 293–99.

Parnetti, L.; Bottiglieri, T.; and Lowenthal, D. "Role of Homocysteine in aging." *Aging Clinical Experimental Research* 1997, 9: 241–57.

Stramentinoli, G.; Gualano, M.; Catto, E.; Algeri S. "Tissue Levels of S-Adenosylmethionine in Aging Rats." *Journal of Gerontology,* July 1977, 32 (4): 392–94.

Surtees, R., and Hyland, K. "Cerebrospinal Fluid Concentrations of S-Adenosylmethionine, Methionine, and 5-Methyltetrahydrofolate in a Reference Population: Cerebrospinal Fluid S-Adenosylmethionine Declines with Age in Humans." *Biochemical Medicine & Metabolic Biology,* October 1990, 44 (2): 192–99.

Varela-Morrieras, G.; Perez-Olleros, L.; Garcia-Cuevas, M.; et al. "Effects of Aging on Folate Metabolism in Rats Fed a Long-Term Folate-Deficient Diet." *International Journal of Vitamin & Nutrition Research* 1994, 64 (4): 294–99.

DEPRESSION

Arana, G. W., and Hyman, S. E. "Antidepressant Drugs," in: *Handbook of Psychiatric Drug Therapy,* 2d ed. Boston: Little, Brown and Company, 1991, 38–78.

Beekman, A. T.; Deeg, D. J.; Van Tilburg, T.; et al. "Major and minor depression in later life: a study of prevalence and risk factors." *Journal of Affective Disorders* 1995, 36: 65–75.

Berney, T. P.; Bhate, S. R.; Kolvin, I.; et al. "The context of childhood depression: The Newcastle Childhood Depression Project." *British Journal of Psychiatry* 1991, 159 (11): 28–35.

Bottiglieri, T. "Folate, Vitamin B$_{12}$ and Neuropsychiatric Disorders." *Nutrition Reviews* 1997, 54: 382–90.

Cross-National Collaborative Group. "The changing rate of major depression: cross-national comparisons." *JAMA* 1992, 268: 3098–3105.

D/ART. "Depression: Define it. Defeat it. Information About D/ART and Depressive Disorders." Rockville, MD: National Institute of Mental Health, March 25, 1992.

D/ART. "The Effects of Depression in the Workplace." Rockville, MD: National Institute of Mental Health.

D/ART. "Facts About Depression." Rockville, MD: National Institute of Mental Health.

Glass, R. M. "Treating depression as a recurrent or chronic disease." *JAMA,* January 6, 1999, 281 (1).

Gold, P. W.; Goodwin, F. K.; and Chrousos, & G. P. "Clinical and biochemical manifestations of depression: relation to the neurobiology of stress." *New England Journal of Medicine* 1988, 117: 413–20.

Goodnick, P. J., and Sandoval, R. "Psychotropic treatment of chronic fatigue syndrome and related disorders." *Journal of Clinical Psychiatry* 1993, 54 (1): 13–20.

Greenberg, P. E.; Stiglin, L. E.; Finkelstein, S. N.; and Berndt, E. R. "Depression: a neglected major illness." *Journal of Clinical Psychiatry* 1993, 54: 419–24.

Greenberg, P. E.; Stiglin, L. E.; Finkelstein, S. N.; and Berndt, E. R. "The economic burden of depression in 1990." *Journal of Clinical Psychiatry* 1993, 54: 405–18.

Gruber, A. J.; Hudson, J. L.; and Pope, H. G., Jr. "The management of treatment-resistant depression in disorders on the interface of psychiatry and medicine: fibromyalgia, chronic fatigue syndrome, migraine, irritable bowel syndrome, atypical facial pain, and premenstrual dysphoric disorder. *Psychiatric Clinics of North America,* June 1996, 19 (2): 361–69.

Hirschfeld, R. M. A.; Keller, M. B.; and Panico, S. "The National Depressive and Manic-Depressive Association Consensus Statement on the Undertreatment of Depression." *JAMA* 1997, 277: 333–40.

Judd, L. L. "The clinical course of unipolar major depressive disorders." *Archives of General Psychiatry* 1997, 54: 989–91.

Katon, E.; Von Kroff, M.; Lin, E.; et al. "Adequacy and duration of antidepressant treatment in primary care." *Medical Care* 1992, 30 (1): 67–76.

Katon, W., and Schulberg, H. "Epidemiology of depression in primary care." *General Hospital Psychiatry* 1992, 14: 237–47.

Kendler, S. K.; Kessler, R. C.; Walters, E. E.; et al. "Stressful life events, genetic liability, and onset of an episode of major depression in women." *American Journal of Psychiatry* 1995, 152: 833–42.

Kupfer, D. J. "Long-term treatment of depression." *Journal of Clinical Psychiatry* 1992, 52 (5): 28–34.

Lebowitz, Barry D.; Pearson, Jane L.; Schneider, Lon S.; et al. "Diagnosis and Treatment of Depression in Late Life: Consensus Statement Update." *JAMA* 1997, 278 (14): 1186–90.

Murphy, J. M. "What happens to depressed men?" *Harvard Review of Psychiatry* 1995, 3: 47–49.

Murray, C. J. L., and Lopez, A. D. "Global mortality, disability, and the contribution of risk factors: Global Burden of Disease Study." *Lancet* 1997, 349: 1436–42.

Musselman, D. L.; Evans, D. L.; and Nemeroff, C. B. "The relationship of depression to cardiovascular disease." *Archives of General Psychiatry* 1998, 55: 580–92.

Nierenberg, A. A., and Cole, J. D. "Antidepressant adverse drug reactions." *Journal of Clinical Psychiatry* 1991, 52: 640–47.

NIH Consensus Development Panel on Depression in Late Life. "Diagnosis and treatment of depression in late life." *JAMA* 1992, 268: 1018–24.

NIMH Office of Scientific Information. "Number of U.S. Adults (in Millions) with Mental Disorders, 1990." Rockville, MD: National Institute of Mental Health, 1998.

Patterson, L. E. "Strategies for improving medication compliance." *Essential Psychopharmacology* 1996, 1 (1): 70–79.

Pennix, B. W. J. H.; Guralnick, J. M.; Ferrucci, L.; et al. "Depressive symptoms and physical decline in community-dwelling older persons." *JAMA* 1998, 279: 1720–26.

Post, R. M. "Transduction of psychosocial stress into the neurobiology of recurrent affective disorder." *American Journal of Psychiatry* 1992, 149: 999–1009.

Rickels, K., and Schweizer, E. "Clinical overview of serotonin reuptake inhibitors." *Journal of Clinical Psychiatry* 1990, 51 (B): 9–12.

Roose, S. P. "Methodological issues in the diagnosis and study of refractory depression, in: Roose, S. P., and Glassman, A. H., eds.: *Treatment Strategies for Refractory Repression.* Washington, D.C.: American Psychiatric Press, 1990: 3–9.

Shapiro, S.; Skinner, E. A.; Kessler, L. G.; et al. "Utilization of health and mental health services: Three Epidemiologic Catchment Area Sites." *Archives of General Psychiatry* 1984, 41: 1971–78.

Simon, E. G.; VonKorff, M.; Heiligenstein, J. H.; et al. "Initial antidepressant choice in primary care: Effectiveness and cost of fluoxetine vs. tricyclic antidepressants." *JAMA* 1996, 275: 1897–1902.

Wehr, T. A., and Rosenthal, N. E. "Seasonality and affective illness." *American Journal of Psychiatry* 1989, 146: 829–39.

Wells, K. B.; Stewart, A.; Hays, R. D.; et al. "The functioning and well-being of depressed patients: Results from the Medical Outcomes Study." *JAMA* 1989, 262: 914–19.

ARTHRITIS

Bassleer, C.; Gysen, P.; Bassler, R.; et al. "Proteoglycans Synthesized by Human Chondrocytes Cultivated in Clusters." *American Journal of Medicine,* November 1987, 83 (5A): 25–28.

Bassleer, C. T.; Henrotin, Y. E.; Regnister, J. L.; and Franchimont, P. P. "Effects of Tiaprofenic Acid and Acetylsalicylic Acid on Human Articular Chondrocytes in 3-Dimensional Culture." *Journal of Rheumatology,* September 1992, 19 (9): 1433–38.

Brandt, K. "Effects of Nonsteroidal Anti-Inflammatory Drugs on Chondrocyte Metabolism in Vitro and in Vivo." *American Journal of Medicine,* November 1987, 83 (5A): 29–35.

Brandt, K. "Should Osteoarthritis Be Treated with Nonsteroidal Anti-Inflammatory Drugs?" *Rheumatic Diseases Clinics of North America,* August 1992, 19 (3): 697–712.

Bibliography

Cox, M. J.; McDevitt, C. A.; Arnocsky, S. P.; et al. "Changes in the Chondroitin Sulfate-Rich Region of Articular Cartilage Proteoglycans in Experimental Osteoarthritis." *Biochimica et Biophysica Acta,* June 1985, 840 (2): 228–34.

D'Ambrosio, E.; Casa, B.; Bompani, R.; et al. "Glucosamine Sulphate: a controlled clinical investigation in arthrosis." *Pharmatherapeutica* 1981, 2 (8): 504–8.

Dingle, J. T. "Cartilage Maintenance in Osteoarthritis Interaction of Cytokines, NSAID and Prostaglandins in Articular Cartilage Damage and Repair." *Journal of Rheumatology*—Supplements March 1991, 28: 30–37.

Fassbender, H. "Role of Chondrocyle in the Development of Osteoarthritis." *American Journal of Medicine* November 1987, 83 (5A): 17–24.

Floman, Y.; Eyre, D. R.; and Glimcher, M. J. "Induction of Osteoarthritis in the Rabbit Knee Joint: Biochemical Studies on the Articular Cartilage." *Clinical Orthopaedics & Related Research,* March-April 1980, (147): 278–86.

Karube, S., and Shoji, H. "Compositional changes of glycosaminoglycans of the human menisci with age and degenerative joint disease." *Nippon Seikeigeka Gakkai Zasshi—Journal of the Japanese Orthopedic Association,* January 1982, 56 (1): 51–57.

Lewandowski, B.; Bernacka, K.; Cylwik, B.; et al. "Piroxicam and Poststeroidal Damage of Articular Cartilage." *Roczniki Akademii Medjznej W Bialymstoku* 1995, 40 (2): 396–408.

Lopes, V. A. "Double-blind clinical evaluation of the relative efficacy of ibuprofen and glucosamine sulphate in the management of osteoarthrosis of the knee in out-patients." *Current Medical Research & Opinion* 1982, 8 (3): 145–49.

Malemud, C.; Shuckett, J. R.; and Goldberg, V. M. "Changes in proteoglycans of human osteoarthritic cartilage maintained in explant culture: Implications for understanding repair in osteoarthritis." *Scandinavian Journal of Rheumatology*—Supplement 1988, 77: 7–12.

Rainsford, K. D. "Mechanisms of NSAIDs on Joint Destruction in Osteoarthritis." *Agents and Actions—Supplements* 1993, 44: 39–42.

SAM-E AND THE LIVER

Angelico, M., Gandin, C.; Nistri, A.; et al. "Oral S-adenosyl-L-methionine (SAMe) administration enhances bile salt conjugation with taurine in patients with liver cirrhosis." *Scandinavian Journal of Clinical & Laboratory Investigation* Oct. 1994; 54 (6): 459–64.

Barak, A. J.; Beckenhauer, E. C.; Tuma, D.J.; and Badakhsh, S. "Effects of prolonged ethanol feeding on methionine metabolism in rat liver." *Biochemistry and Cell Biology,* March 1987, 65 (3): 230–33.

Cantoni, L.; Maggi, G.; Mononi, G.; and Preti G. "Relations between protidopoiesis and biological transmethylations: action of S-adenosylmethionine on protein crisis in chronic hepatopathies." *Minerva Medica,* May 1975, 66 (33): 1581–9.

Chawla, R. K.; Bonkovsky, H. L.; and Galambos, J. T. "Biochemistry and pharmacology of S-adenosyl-L-methionine and rationale for its use in liver disease." *Drugs* 1990, 40 (3): 98–110.

Duce, A. M.; Ortiz, P.; Cabrero, G.; and Mato, J. M. "S-adenosyl-L-methionine synthetase and phospholipid methyltransferase are inhibited in human cirrhosis." *Hepatology,* January-February 1998, 8 (1): 65–68.

Frezza, M.; Centini, G.; Cammareri, G.; et al. "S-adenosylmethionine for the Treatment of Intrahepatic Cholestasis of Pregnancy: Results of a Controlled Clinical Trial." *Hepato-gastrointerology* 1990, Supp. 11:122–25.

Frezza, M.; Pozzato, G.; Chiesa, L.; et al. "Reversal of intrahepatic cholestasis of pregnancy in women after high-dose S-adenosylmethionine administration." *Hepatology* 1984, 4: 274–78.

Friedel, H. A.; Goa, K. L.; and Benfield, P. "S-adenosyl-L-methionine: a review of its therapeutic potential in liver dysfunction and affective disorders in relation to its physiological role in cell metabolism." *Drugs* 1989, 38: 389–416.

Ideo, G. "S-adenosylmethionine: plasma levels in hepatic cirrhosis and preliminary results of its clinical use in hepatology: double-blind study." *Minerva Medica,* May 1975, 66 (33): 1581–9.

Kakimoto, H.; Kawata, S.; Imaim, Y.; et al. "Changes in lipid composition of erythrocyte membranes with administration of S-adenosyl-L-methionine in chronic liver disease." *Gastroenterologia Japonica,* August 1992, 27 (4): 508–13.

Labo, G.; Miglio, F. D.; D'Ambro, A.; et al. "Double-blind polycentric study of the action of S-adenosylmethionine in hepatic cirrhosis." *Minerva Medica,* May 1975, 66 (33): 1590–4.

Lieber, C. S.; Casini, A.; DeCarli, L. M.; et al. "S-adenosyl-L-methionine attenuates alcohol-induced liver injury in the baboon." *Hepatology* 1990, 11: 165–72.

Lieber, C. S., and Williams, R. "Recent advances in the treatment of liver diseases." *Drugs* 1990, 40 (3): 1–38.

Loguercio, C.; Nardi, G.; Argenzio, F.; et al. "Effect of S-adenosyl-L-methionine administration on red blood cell cysteine and glutathione levels in alcoholic patients with and without liver disease." *Alcohol & Alcoholism,* September 1994, 29 (5): 597–604.

Micali, M.; Chiti, D.; and Balestra, V. "Double-blind controlled clinical trial of SAMe administered orally in chronic liver diseases." *Current Therapeutic Research* 1983, 33: 1004–13.

Miglio, E.; Stefanini, G. F.; Corazza, G. R.; et al. "Double-blind studies of the therapeutic action of S-adenosylmethionine (SAMe) in oral administration in liver cirrhosis and other chronic hepatitides." *Minerva Medica,* May 1995, 66 (33): 1595–99.

Nicastri, P. L.; Diaferia, A.; Tartagni, M.; Loizzi, P.; and Fanelli, M. "A randomised placebo-controlled trial of ursodeoxycholic acid and S-adenosylmethionine in the treatment of intrahepatic cholestasis of pregnancy." *British Journal of Obstetrics & Gynaecology* 1998, 105(11): 1205–7.

Osman, E.; Owen, J. S.; and Burroughs, A. K. "S-adenosyl-L-methionine: a new therapeutic agent in liver disease? *Alimentary Pharmacological Therapy* 1993, 7: 21–28.

Pisi, E., and Marchesini, G. "Mechanisms and consequences of the impaired trans-sulphuration pathway in liver disease: Part II. Clinical consequences and potential for pharmacological intervention in cirrhosis." *Drugs* 1990, 40 (3): 65–72.

Shield, M. J. "Anti-Inflammatory Drugs and Their Effects on Cartilage Synthesis and Renal Function." *European Journal of Rheumatology & Inflammation* 1993, 13 (1): 7–16.

Vendemiale, G.; Altomare, E.; Trizio, T.; et al. "Effects of oral S-adenosyl-L-methionine on hepatic glutathione in patients with liver disease." *Scandinavian Journal of Gastroenterology* 1989, 24: 407–15.

SAM-E

Castagna, A.; Le Grazie, C.; Giulidori, P.; Bottiglieri, T.; and Lazzarin, A. "Deficiency of CSF S-adenosylmethionine (SAMe) and glutathione in HIV infected patients: the effect of parenteral treatment with SAMe." *Neurology* 1995, 45: 1678–83.

Chiang, P. K.; Gordon, R. K.; Tal, J.; et al. "S-Adeno-sylmethionine and methylation." *Federation of the American Society of Experimental Biology Journal* 1996, 10: 471–80.

Cozens, D. D., et al. "Reproductive Toxicity Studies of Ademe-tionine." *Arzneimittel-Forschung,* November 1988, 38 (11): 1625–29.

Evans, P. J.; Whiteman, M.; Tredger, J. M.; and Halliwell, B. "Antioxidant properties of S-adenosyl-L-methionine: a proposed addition to organ storage fluids." *Free Radicals in Biology and Medicine* 1997, 23(7): 1002–8.

Giulidori, P.; Cortellaro, M.; Moreo, G.; and Stramentinoli, G. "Pharmacokinetics of S-adenosyl-L-methionine in healthy volunteers." *European Journal of Clinical Pharmacology* 1984, 227: 119–21.

Lo Russo, A.; Monaco, M.; Pani, A.; et al. "Efficacy of

S-adenosyl-L-methionine in relieving psychological distress associated with detoxification in opiate abusers." *Current Therapeutic Research* 1994, 55: 905–13.

Loehrer, F. M.; Angst, C. P.; Haefeli, W. E.; et al. "Low whole-blood S-adenosylmethionine and correlation with 5-methyltetrahydrofolate and homocysteine in coronary artery disease." *Arteriosclerosis and Thrombosis Biology* 1996, 16: 727–33.

Shekim, W. O.; Antun, F.; Hanna, G. L.; et al. "S-adenosyl-L-methionine (SAM) in adults with ADHD, RS: preliminary results from an open trial." *Psychopharmacology Bulletin* 1990, 26 (2): 249–53.

Yatsugi, S.; Yamamoto, T.; Ohno, M.; and Ueki, S. "Effect of S-adenosyl-L-methionine on impairment of working memory induced in rats by cerebral ischemia and scopolamine." *European Journal of Pharmacology* 1989, 166: 231–39.

SAM-E AND FIBROMYALGIA

Buchwald, D. "Fibromyalgia and chronic fatigue syndrome: similarities and differences." *Rheumatic Diseases Clinics of North America,* May 1996, 22 (2): 219–43.

Di Benedetto, P.; Iona, L. G.; and Zidarich, V. "Clinical evaluation of S-adenosyl-L-methionine versus transcutaneous electrical nerve stimulation in primary fibromyalgia." *Current Therapeutic Research* 1993, 53: 222–29

Hudson, J. I., and Pope, H. G., Jr. "The relationship between fibromyalgia and major depressive disorder." *Rheumatic Diseases Clinics of North America,* May 1996, 22 (2): 285–303.

Jacobsen, S.; Danneskiold-Samsoe, B.; and Anderson, R. B. "Oral S-adenosylmethionine in primary fibromyalgia:

double-blind clinical evaluation." *Scandinavian Journal of Rheumatology* 1991, 20 (4): 294–302

Tavoni, A.; Vitali, C.; Bonbardieri, S.; and Pasero, G. "Evaluation of S-Adenosylmethionine in Primary Fibromyalgia: A Double-Blind Cross-over Study." *American Journal of Medicine,* November 1987, 83 (5A): 107–10.

Volkman, H.; Norregaard, J.; Jacobson, S.; et al. "Double-blind, placebo-controlled crossover study of intravenous S-adenosyl-L-methionine in patients with fibromyalgia." *Scandinavian Journal of Rheumatology* 1997, 26 (3): 206–11.